Sleep
to be Sexy
Smart
and Slim

"This thoughtful book is a must read!"
　　　　—Julie Silver, M.D., Assistant Professor, Harvard Medical
　　　　School, and author of *Super Healing* and *After Cancer
　　　　Treatment: Heal Faster, Better, Stronger*

"The authors have done a masterful job of bringing together proven advice from the leading experts to help us all get the sleep we need to be at our best physically and mentally."
　　　　—Diane Heavin, Founder of Curves International and
　　　　Publisher of *diane* magazine

"Sleep is not a luxury—it is essential."
　　　　—Jodi A. Mindell, Ph.D., Associate Director of the Sleep
　　　　Center at the Children's Hospital of Philadelphia and
　　　　author of *Sleep Deprived No More: From Pregnancy to
　　　　Early Motherhood*

"Now you AND your child can get a good night's sleep!"
　　　　—Karen Cicero, Special Projects Editor, *Parents* magazine

"Continued development of societal systems that operate 24 hours a day, seven days a week, with an increasing emphasis on cognitive capability, has created a lifestyle...that is, paradoxically, cognitively incapacitating...because [the] biological forces that require us to sleep also appear to be critical to waking cognitive capability."
　　　　—David Dinges, Ph.D., recent president of the World
　　　　Federation of Sleep Research and Sleep Medicine
　　　　Societies

Sleep

to be Sexy

Smart

and Slim

Get the Best Sleep of Your Life
Tonight and *Every Night*

Ellen Michaud with Julie Bain
Health Director, Reader's Digest Magazine

FOREWORD BY Mary Susan Esther, M.D.
The Sleep Center at SouthPark
Charlotte Eye Ear Nose and Throat Associates
Charlotte, North Carolina
PRESIDENT, AMERICAN ACADEMY OF SLEEP MEDICINE

Reader's

The Reader's Digest Association, Inc.

Pleasantville, New York/Montreal/London/Sydney

U.S. Project Editor Barbara Booth
Canadian Project Editor Pamela Chichinskas
Australian Project Editor Annette Carter
Copy Editor Kim Casey
Associate Art Director George McKeon
Illustrator Heather Holbrook
Cover Designer Jennifer Tokarski
Project Production Coordinator Wayne Morrison
Indexer Andrea Chesman
Executive Editor, Trade Publishing Dolores York
Production Manager Elizabeth Dinda
Vice President, U.S. Operations Michael Braunschweiger
Associate Publisher Rosanne McManus
President and Publisher, Trade Publishing Harold Clarke

Library of Congress Cataloging-in-Publication Data:
Michaud, Ellen.
  Sleep to be sexy, smart, and slim : how to get the best sleep of your life
tonight and every night / Ellen Michaud with Julie Bain.
      p. cm.
  Includes bibliographical references and index.
  ISBN 0-7621-0931-9 (978-0-7621-0931-9 : alk. paper)
  1. Sleep. 2. Women--Health and hygiene. 3. Insomnia--Prevention. I. Bain, Julie. II. Title.
  RA786.M53 2008
  613.7'9--dc22
                                          2007046119

We are committed to both the quality of our products and the service we provide
to our customers. We value your comments, so please feel free to contact us.

The Reader's Digest Association, Inc.
Adult Trade Publishing
Reader's Digest Road
Pleasantville, NY 10570-7000

For more Reader's Digest products and information, visit our website:
www.rd.com (in the United States)
www.readersdigest.ca (in Canada)
www.readersdigest.com.au (in Australia)
www.readersdigest.co.uk (in the United Kingdom)

The names of sleepless women throughout this book
have been changed to protect their privacy.

NOTE TO OUR READERS
This is a reference volume only. The information in this book should not be
substituted for, or used to alter, medical therapy without your doctor's advice.
For a specific health problem, consult your physician for guidance. The Reader's Digest
Association, Inc., assumes no responsibility or liability for any injuries, damages, or losses
incurred during the use of, or as a result of, following this information.

Printed in the United States of America

1 3 5 7 9 10 8 6 4 2

Contents

Foreword

Nearly 25 years ago, while holding a squalling infant who hadn't closed his eyes in more than 24 hours, or so it seemed at the time, it became apparent to me that I had been underestimating the importance of sleep.

Today common sense tells us that good sleep is essential for good health—and science is now showing us exactly how.

Researchers have determined that insufficient sleep can cause serious medical problems—high blood pressure, diabetes, obesity, and depression, to begin with. They've also found that an inability to fall asleep or to maintain sleep can be an indicator of many underlying medical problems. And they've discovered, too, that insufficient sleep, whether by choice or of necessity, is a leading cause of accidents in today's world.

Perhaps one of the most significant problems has been that for a long time scientists believed sleep to be a "passive" state rather than a dynamic brain activity, as it is now known. Researchers have since demonstrated that the dreaming brain is far from "quiet" and can have more blood flow than in wakeful states. In fact, we now know that sleep is a complicated

"This marvelous book presents a straightforward approach toward what needs to happen to obtain a good night's sleep."

physiological process whose delicate balance is easily disrupted.

As with dietary habits, it is sleep "habits" that are often critical. For the past decade research has shown that a behavioral approach to insomnia is effective and lasting if it is seriously undertaken and followed systematically.

While it is often easier to look to various medications for sleep assistance, it is in the examining and making of changes to your sleep habits where you can really make the difference. And having an understanding of what is involved in developing a healthy sleep pattern is a first, critical step.

Sleep to be Sexy, Smart, and Slim is an impressive guide that explores not only sleep habits but also sleep disorders and their treatments. The authors explain the complexities of sleep and give practical solutions to common problems. Everything from the importance of limiting caffeine intake and the real effects of alcohol on sleep to "turning off the BlackBerry" is explored, along with a discussion of complicated sleep physiology, the effects of sleep on diet, and the hormonal effects of sleep debt.

It is one book that will, thankfully, put us all to sleep.

—Mary S. Esther, M.D.
The Sleep Center at SouthPark
Charlotte Eye Ear Nose and Throat Associates
Charlotte, North Carolina
PRESIDENT, AMERICAN ACADEMY OF SLEEP MEDICINE

Introduction

You've done low-carb, high-protein. High-carb, low-protein. High-carb, high-fiber, no dairy. Plus, you've had intimate relationships with Dr. Atkins, Jenny Craig, Dr. Phil, and the Duchess of York.

But you still can't budge that last 10 pounds off your hips, and if you don't watch every latte that slides down your throat, that 5 pounds you struggled so hard to lose last summer will creep right back.

But what if your problem isn't your diet? What if you are, in fact, eating healthfully and exercising the way your fitness trainer intended? What if it isn't a question of willpower, discipline, and counting calories?

What if the problem is your *sleep?*

Until the last couple of decades or so, scientists hadn't seriously looked at sleep. But now that they have the time, the money, and the technology to investigate what they've been missing out on each night, there's been one amazing discovery after another.

For one thing, they've discovered that while you're asleep, your brain runs a checklist that would put NASA to shame. Every single system is being fine-tuned, reset, cleaned up, and restored to optimal operating mode by an army of molecular troubleshooters.

New things you've learned are being processed, memories are being organized and stored, and the immune system is building a new contingent of natural killer cells to fight off battalions of infectious agents and cancers. Growth hormone is being produced as well to repair damaged tissue (in adults) or build new tissue (in children) and to directly block the corrosive effects of stress. When all these molecular activities take place on schedule during a good night's sleep, you're in peak operating condition when your eyes snap open the next morning.

When these activities don't take place, you not only feel groggy, none of your systems are firing on all cylinders. You don't think straight, make good decisions, remember where you parked the car, or feel like making love.

Sadly, studies also show that when your body doesn't get enough sleep for the usual repair and maintenance, your mood is flat, there's no joy in life, a single stressor like a flat tire will cause you to freak out, and the resulting chemical glitches will put you on the fast track for heart disease, stroke, diabetes, and obesity.

Yeah, you read that right. Obesity. Unfortunately, tossing and turning lowers levels of leptin, the hormone that causes you to feel full, while increasing levels of ghrelin, the hormone that makes you feel hungry.

Think that can't have an effect? An amazing study of 68,000 women conducted at Harvard Medical School reveals that women who sleep five hours a night are 32 percent more likely to gain 30 pounds or more as they get older than women who sleep seven hours or more.

Survival in a 24/7 Culture

So why aren't we sleeping? Jobs, kids, partners, allergies, parents, depression—some nights it seems as though there's one obstacle after another. But after interviewing more than 30 of the world's most brilliant sleep researchers, we've found that just about every one of us is losing sleep because we live in a 24/7 culture.

Not that we want to change it. God forbid. What on earth would we do if we couldn't download a movie at 1:00 A.M. or call the Bank of America's call center in Hyderabad, India, at 2:00 A.M.?

Life would be tough. BlackBerries, cell phones, and other interactive technologies keep us informed, connected, updated, and available around the clock. We can check on our children, conference with colleagues, hear from suppliers, track shipments, order pizza, download a movie, upload a report, play solitaire, and schedule a flight to L.A. at any time of the day or night.

And it's good for the economy, right? Millions of jobs have been created for the night workers who serve us. From the guy who delivers that 11:00 P.M. pizza we ordered to the supplier who has his or her people working in three shifts around the clock; from the truck driver who drives all night to get a package on our desk by 9:00 A.M. to the ER doctor who sews us back together when we fall asleep at the wheel, a whopping 25 million people in the United States have created an entire nation of people who work at night.

But as David Dinges, Ph.D., recent president of the World Federation of Sleep Research and Sleep Medicine Societies, points out, our stubborn insistence on finding ways to stay awake at all hours of the night has actually led us to break through the built-in genetic safety barriers that have kept us from getting into trouble.

We're genetically primed to get sleepy after it gets dark, but electric lights and a cup of coffee allow us to override that cue and keep going. We're genetically primed to wake when it gets light, but intense artificial lighting at night and room-darkening shades in the morning will allow us to ignore that cue, too.

And when our minds are so exhausted we lose our cell phones, keys, and anything else that's not permanently attached to our bodies, instead of taking the hint and taking a nap, 67 percent of us ignore our brain's pleas for sleep, knock back a cup of coffee or a different caffeinated drink, and just keep going.

The thing is, not only is our propensity for overriding genetic cues leading us down the path to being fat, forgetful, diabetic, sexless, and prone to heart disease and cancer, it's also sabotaging our ability to function in that same 24/7 culture.

How can we analyze competitive data for the businesses that employ us if we can't focus on it long enough to compare one set of numbers with another?

How can we build the next new-new thing if our brain cells are too worn out to dream it up?

How can we elect leaders who will guide us safely through global minefields if we can't focus our attention on candidates long enough to strip away the convoluted "spin" that characterizes so much of American politics?

How can we learn new systems and technologies if we're falling asleep over our keyboards?

How can we invent those same systems and technologies if we haven't the energy to send our intellect soaring into the deep space of our imagination?

How can we think, analyze, integrate, learn, and strategize without taking the time to repair, restructure, and renew the very basic neurobiology that has allowed us to create the 24/7 culture?

As Dr. Dinges recently told a world conference of sleep researchers, "Continued development of societal systems that operate 24 hours a day, seven days a week, with an increasing emphasis on cognitive capability, has created a lifestyle for hundreds of millions of people around the globe that is, paradoxically, cognitively incapacitating and potentially unhealthy because [the] biological forces that require us to sleep also appear to be critical to waking cognitive capability and health maintenance."

In other words, by not getting enough sleep, we're destroying the very capabilities we need to survive.

This book will help you turn that around.

—Ellen Michaud
sleep.rd.com

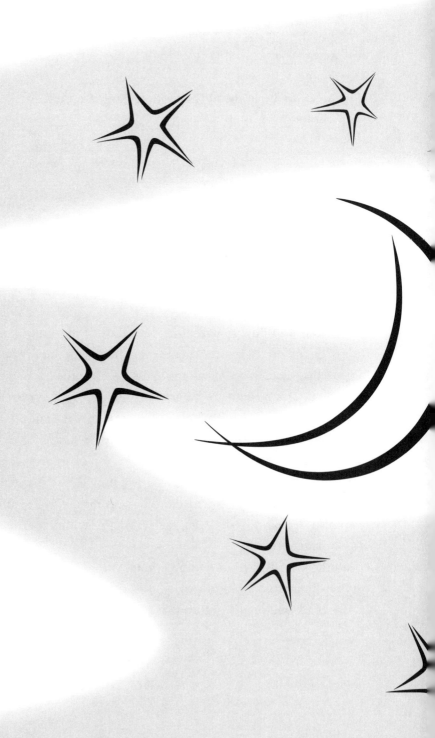

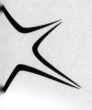

Part I

Do You
Have a
Sleep
Problem?

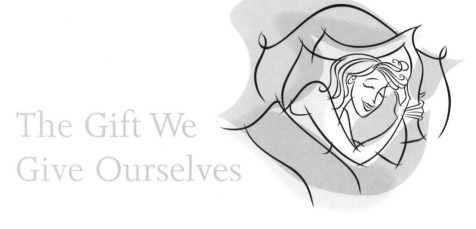

The Gift We Give Ourselves

Forty-four-year-old Sarah Brigham smiled down at the triple chocolate birthday cake her coworkers had just put on the conference table. The next day was her birthday, and she was ready to celebrate.

Her boss stepped in beside her as she sliced the cake. He knew she'd

By age 50 **only 32 percent** of **women** get a **good night's sleep** even a few nights **a month.**

been working around the clock for months on a new launch, and he was particularly appreciative of the fact that despite having two kids at home—one in high school, the other an active sixth-grader—she'd worked 10- to 12-hour days and hadn't taken a personal or vacation day in months. But she was taking off on her birthday, and he was curious. "So what are you going to do tomorrow?" he asked, as he accepted a plate.

Sara lifted an eyebrow and, for a moment, looked less like a project manager and more like a three-year-old.

"Sleep!" she said gleefully.

The Trend toward Sleep Deprivation

Somewhere in the recent past, sleep became a gift that we give ourselves only on special occasions such as Mother's Day or a birthday.

Ten years ago at least 38 percent of us slept eight hours a night, which, depending on personal biology and life stage, is what most of us need. Five years ago that number dropped to 30 percent. Two years ago it was down to 26. Now, well, let's just say that sleep researchers are aghast at the low numbers they are gleaning from their latest surveys.

What even these early numbers mean, however, is clear: More than 75 percent of us are not getting enough sleep, and only 60 percent of us get a good night's sleep a few nights a week or less.

Fortunately, that can change. But the first step toward getting a good night's sleep is to find out exactly how sleep deprived you really are. So take the quiz "How Bad Is It?" which begins on page 6, and let's take a look.

EARLY WARNING SIGNS

"Even before sleep problems show themselves as weight gain, lack of interest in sex, a flattened emotional response, illness, or forgetfulness, you'll have problems paying attention, sustaining attention, and falling asleep while reading or driving," says researcher David F. Dinges, Ph.D., recent president of the World Federation of Sleep Research and Sleep Medicine Societies.

The moment you realize you're doing any of those things, says Dr. Dinges, it's time to rethink priorities and move sleep to the top of your to-do list. And in today's world, that's easier said than done.

WHO'S UP?

Twenty million women are tossing and turning on a nightly basis. Here's a sampling of who's up, along with why, what they do about it, and what they are up against.

- 60 percent of women get a good night's sleep only a couple of times a week.

- 74 percent of stay-at-home moms can't sleep.

- 72 percent of working moms can't sleep.

- 68 percent of single working women can't sleep.

- 80 percent are kept up by worrying about things.

- 43 percent say daytime sleepiness interferes with daily activities like jobs and child care.

- 80 percent of sleep-deprived women just suck it up and go on with their daily activities.

- 67 percent use a caffeinated beverage to help.

- 33 percent have given up sex.

- 25 percent have recently driven while drowsy.

- 10 percent have driven while drowsy with a child in the car.

- 37 percent have fallen asleep at the wheel.

Sources:
1. The National Sleep Foundation.
2. The National Highway Safety Administration.

How Bad Is It?

The Epworth Sleepiness Scale, developed by Dr. Murray Johns of Epworth Hospital in Melbourne, Australia, is a standard used by sleep specialists to judge a person's level of daytime sleepiness. To find out your level, simply circle the answers below that answer the question "What are the chances you'll doze off in these situations?"

❏ **Sitting and reading**

__ 0 None

__ 1 Slight

__ 2 Moderate

__ 3 High

❏ **Watching TV**

__ 0 None

__ 1 Slight

__ 2 Moderate

__ 3 High

❏ **Sitting inactively in a public place, such as a theater or a meeting**

__ 0 None

__ 1 Slight

__ 2 Moderate

__ 3 High

❏ **As a passenger in a car for an hour without a break**

__ 0 None

__ 1 Slight

__ 2 Moderate

__ 3 High

❏ **Lying down to rest in the afternoon**

__ 0 None

__ 1 Slight

__ 2 Moderate

__ 3 High

❏ **Sitting and talking to someone**

___ 0 None

___ 1 Slight

___ 2 Moderate

___ 3 High

❏ **Sitting quietly after a lunch (without alcohol)**

___ 0 None

___ 1 Slight

___ 2 Moderate

___ 3 High

❏ **In a car while stopped for a few minutes in traffic**

___ 0 None

___ 1 Slight

___ 2 Moderate

___ 3 High

Now total up your score. Here's what we think it means:

❏ If you tallied less than 8 points on our sleep quiz, you're in good shape. You probably get a full eight hours of slumber every night, bounce out of bed at 5:00 A.M., and are ready to charge out the door an hour later.

❏ If you tallied 8 to 11 points on our sleep quiz, you experience mild sleepiness that may not have gotten you into trouble yet, but you're clearly cruising down the wrong road. Have you been gaining weight?

❏ If you tallied 12 to 15 points, we're guessing that you get maybe five or six hours of sleep a night. You try to catch up on weekends, but Monday mornings are a bear. If there weren't a Starbucks on the way to work, you'd be in deep trouble.

❏ If you tallied 16 to 24 points, you get so little sleep that you shouldn't be behind the wheel of a car, balancing your checkbook, or figuring out your income tax. We have concerns for you, girl.

What's Your Sleep Style?

Okay. Now that you've realized how sleepy you are, you're probably ready to make some changes. But this book is overflowing with so many sleep strategies, we thought you'd like a little help figuring out where to start.

So we asked Philadelphia psychologist Suzanne Zoglio, Ph.D., to develop a quiz that will reveal your sleep style. Once you know your type, you can determine which actions to take next.

Take the One-Minute Quiz

Read each statement that follows and decide how frequently it is true for you. Take stock of your answers by following the instructions on the next page. Then put it all together and find your style. Are you a Comfort Queen? A Strong Starter? Other? Turn to page 10 and find out.

Always	Often	Seldom	Never
4	3	2	0

1. __ When others are talking, your mind wanders off.

2. __ You make the same resolutions over and over.

3. __ If you get a headache, you don't hesitate to take an aspirin ASAP.

4. __ If you could wear your slippers to work, you would.

5. __ "I don't have the time" could be your mantra.

6. __ You are a champion multitasker.

7. __ After a hard day a glass of wine is your favorite relaxer.

8. __ You could happily sit on a beach for an hour or more.

9. __ You want to change something but can't seem to make it happen.

10. __ If you lose a button, a safety pin will do…for the life of the jacket.

11. __ People often ask you for help.

12. __ If stuck in traffic, you're likely to listen to music or daydream.

13. __ A hotel room with a feather bed is your kind of place.

14. __ You wish you had someone to advise and encourage you.

15. __ A lavender-scented candle would be a perfect gift for you.

Scoring

A. Total your responses to items 2, 9, and 14. This is your **Strong Starter** score:__

B. Total your responses to items 3, 7, and 10. This is your **Quick Fixer** score:__

C. Total your responses to items 4, 13, and 15. This is your **Comfort Queen** score:__

D. Total your responses to items 1, 8, and 12. This is your **Daydreamer** score:__

E. Total your responses to items 5, 6, and 11. This is your **BlackBerry Babe** score:__

Now, using your highest score(s), read the matching style description(s) below.

A. Strong Starter. You want to grow, regularly get psyched for change, but lose steam before you meet your goals. Not quite sure why you can't stick to a plan, you'd probably welcome some sound advice and some encouragement. Check out the sleep strategies involving doctors and/or professional advice first.

B. Quick Fixer. Practical and impatient with a low tolerance for suffering, you are likely to try anything that's fast, simple, and yields quick results, even if they are short term. Sleep strategies you should consider first include sleep medication, waking at the same time every day, and low-fat cookies before bed.

C. Comfort Queen. If it feels good, smells good, or tastes good, bring it on! You can luxuriate for an hour in a warm bubble bath but you wouldn't be caught dead in a cold, smelly gym. The sleep strategies that will get you started include ones that modify your environment—silk sheets, hot soaks, and cool socks to start.

D. Daydreamer. While others need to be physically moving, actively engaged, or entertained, you seem quite comfortable alone with your thoughts. Patient, calm, and introspective, you're likely to find the serene sleep strategies—like mental imagery, prayer, and meditation—to be just your cup of tea.

E. BlackBerry Babe. With the middle name "24/7," what can you expect? You're amazing, and everyone knows it. You're never out of contact, seldom say no, and regularly suffer from a mind in overdrive. For you sleep remedies begin with setting boundaries, managing electronics, online therapy, and clarifying your priorities.

What's It All Mean?

Now that you've established your style, turn to Part II, "Surefire Sleep Strategies," to discover your best tips and tricks for getting a good night's sleep. Then, once you're on the path back from the dark side, you can add other strategies—plus any from Part III, "Sleep Saboteurs across the Lifespan"—that may be helpful. Part III includes the most common barriers to sleep, such as kids, restless bed partners, stress, worry, cancer, pregnancy, aging parents, jet lag, and a 24/7 work life.

Sound like your life? Yeah—ours, too.

Part II

Surefire Strategies for Getting a Good Night's Sleep

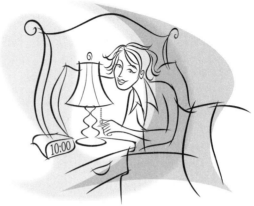

To Sleep, Perchance to Dream…

Sleep is sweet.

Emerging from a warm, cozy nest of pillows after a night of blissfully restorative sleep is heaven. You push back the blankets and everything seems brighter. Unfortunately, that experience doesn't happen as often as it should. Doctors can actually hook us up to a computer and see the neurological chatter on screen while we sleep.

Stress, worry, money, kids— they **all** combine with the **demands** of the **workplace.**

We deserve better. That's why we've asked the very best sleep medicine specialists from across the continent to give us a list of surefire strategies that will help us not only *get* to sleep but also *stay* asleep. Their recommendations are discussed in more depth throughout the following chapters, but we've folded key strategies into a start-now plan that will allow you to begin tinkering with your brain chemistry today. No more tossing and turning. No more middle-of-the-night dialogues with yourself. Here's what to do.

Timing Is All

 When you go to bed and when you get up are keystones to restful, refreshing sleep. Once you learn to synchronize your body's biological clock, your body will know when to sleep and when to be alert.

WAKE AT THE SAME TIME EVERY DAY. A good night's sleep actually starts in the morning. The second your eyes flutter open, light shoots down the optic nerve and into the brain's biological clock. There it stimulates the production of a smorgasbord of hormones that regulate growth, reproduction, eating, sleeping, thinking, remembering—even how you feel from minute to minute.

"Sunlight activates the brain," says Frisca L. Yan-Go, M.D., medical director of the UCLA Sleep Disorders Center. And activating it at the same time every morning synchronizes your body's biological clock. Then your body has a clear direction that at midnight it's supposed to be asleep and at noon it's supposed to be awake.

Wake up at a different time every day and the clock is out of sync. You feel groggy and hungover for hours, and even when you start to feel a bit more alert after that first Starbucks, you really never achieve the mental edge of which you're capable.

HIT THE SHEETS *ONLY* WHEN SLEEPY. No, not just tired. Sleepy, as in your eyes are droopy and you keep losing track of what people are saying to you.

GET UP. Sleeping from 11:30 P.M. until 2:00 A.M., tossing and turning until 4, then sleeping until 6 gives you eight hours in bed but only 4 1/2 hours of sleep. That's a huge mismatch that can actually inhibit your sleep drive and cause insomnia all by itself. To prevent that from exacerbating your sleep issues, when you wake at 2:00 A.M., get up and go read a book in the living room. Being up increases your sleep drive—

which just could make you sleepy enough to actually fall asleep when you return to bed.

One caveat: Don't stay in bed when you're awake. A part of your mind will begin to associate the bed with being awake rather than being asleep. And that can turn on a nasty "I'm-not-going-to-sleep!" anxiety that will rev your engines whenever you get into bed. It's one of the most insidious—and potent—causes of chronic insomnia.

GIVE YOURSELF AN HOUR. The one right before bed. You need it to wind down and transition from the woman-who-can-do-everything into the woman-who-can-sleep. Unfortunately, most women are not giving themselves one single second. According to the 2007 National Sleep Foundation poll, during the hour before bed, around 60 percent of us do household chores, 37 percent take care of children, 36 percent do activities with other family members, 36 percent are on the Internet, and 21 percent do work related to their jobs.

BEWARE SUNDAY NIGHT INSOMNIA. Staying up late on Friday and Saturday nights and sleeping in on Saturday and Sunday mornings is frequently the gift we give ourselves on weekends after a hard week at work. Yet that little gift—small as it is—is enough to screw up our biological clocks. Even if you get to bed early on Sunday night, you will not be ready to sleep, and you will not end up being the happy camper you were expecting come Monday morning.

> "The lifestyle today is too fast and too complicated. We go all day long at a speed of 110 m.p.h. and then expect our bodies to go down to zero when it's time to turn out the light. I just can't do it, and I worry about it before I even get under the covers. I wish I had some sort of sleep routine to get my body ready for bed, but I just don't have one. I guess watching reruns of CSI isn't the answer."
>
> —SUSAN CERVINI

Feather Your Nest

To lull you to sleep, you need to make your bedroom a sensuous haven, adding all the accoutrements of comfort and serenity in a beautiful setting.

BUY A NEW MATTRESS. Don't even try to comparison shop. Every mattress in every store has a different name. And every owner of every mattress shop says that the mattresses in his shop are different—and better—than every other mattress shop on the planet. The truth is that the right mattress for you is the one that you try in your home for 30 days. Find a mattress shop that offers that option, pick out the mattress that you and your partner think is the most comfortable, make sure it has a guarantee, and flash your plastic. Don't worry about coils and foam and luxury toppers. The mattress that allows you to sink into a

DREAM A SLIMMER YOU

How many calories does an extra two hours of sleep burn? Almost 300, reveals a study at Hendrix College in Conway, Arkansas.

Researchers at the college asked 32 summer students to keep diaries noting how much sleep they got and what foods they ate over a three-week period. The first week, students stuck to their normal eating and sleeping schedules so researchers could see their normal routine. The second week, students were asked to sleep an extra two hours a day. The third week, students returned to their normal routine.

When researchers compared the students' diaries after the third week, they found that the students who got an extra two hours of sleep in week 2 ate nearly 300 calories a day less than in week 1. When they returned to their normal sleep-deprived routines in week 3, they ate more food.

deep, natural sleep and wake up in the morning without aches and pains is the one you want. And there's only one way to find out which mattress that is.

BASK IN COMFORT. Buy silky, natural tree-fiber sheets in a soothing color. An exquisitely soft cashmere throw for the bed. A hypoallergenic down comforter. A sunshine silk duvet cover. Pillows, pillows, and more pillows. A roll for behind your neck, a wedge for behind your back, a full-body pillow for when your bed partner is away. Hypoallergenic, of course. And don't forget the teddy bear. No girl can sleep without one.

SPRITZ. A quick spritz of soothing lavender water on your pillows before bed will help calm your exhausted mind.

CHILL BEFORE BED. Lower the temperature of your bedroom before you climb into bed, says Becky Wang-Cheng, M.D., a medical director at Kettering Medical Center in Ohio. Lower temperatures signal your body it's time to sleep. If your bed partner objects, just tell him to bundle up.

SOAK. A hot bath also helps you lower your body's temperature. Yeah, your temperature goes up while you're in the bath, but your body's response to the heat will be to drop your temperature way down low.

SCHEDULE A MASSAGE. "Massage interrupts the neurohormones connected with sleeplessness and almost manually imposes sleep on you," says therapist Belleruth Naparstek, M.S. "If you can't afford a massage, go to a massage school. You can get one there for $15."

GET MEAN. Women aren't used to nurturing themselves or putting themselves first. But sleep is so necessary to health and happiness that you have to do it. If the dog's snoring wakes you up, then put him in another room. If your partner's snoring wakes you up, help him get treatment. If he refuses to cooperate, put him in another room, too.

SHUT THE DRAPES. You sleep better in the dark. If your eyelids flutter open as you move from one stage of sleep to another, even streetlights or a full moon can wake you up.

DITCH THE NIGHT-LIGHTS. You can also get rid of the clock radios with lighted displays. It turns out your brain can misinterpret even such dim lights and wonder if it should wake you up. "Dark inhibits the brain's biological clock," says Dr. Yan-Go. It tells your brain it's time to sleep.

PULL ON SOCKS. There's no solid explanation for it, but studies have found that wearing socks to bed helps you sleep. It may be that warming your feet and legs allows your internal body temperature to drop.

IGNORE THE CLOCK. Turn your clock's face or digital readout away so you can't see it. We wake slightly throughout the night. A glimpse of your clock—and the realization that you have to get up soon—is enough to jolt you out of sleep and keep you out.

SLEEP NAKED. It's easier to adjust your comfort zone with sheets and blankets you can pull up or throw off rather than a long nightgown or a pair of fleece pajamas, says neurologist Charles J. Bae, M.D., a sleep specialist at the Cleveland Clinic Sleep Disorders Center. The idea is to make the adjustment in a way that rouses you from sleep the least.

"I've gotten to the point that I don't bother to turn in until 3:00 A.M. because it's too hard for me to get to sleep. Instead, I clean up the kitchen, do laundry, and go through mail until I simply can't keep my eyes open. Yes, I still get up at 8 with the rest of the world; I'm just not functioning until 10. I need help!"
—JOCELYN PHILLIPS

Simplify Your Life

Look over your priorities and see what is really important to your work, your family, and your life. Pare down everything else.

DUMP THE 24/7 STUFF. On call to managers, kids, husbands, neighbors, friends, and sometimes even complete strangers who break down on the road, most of us are on the move from the second we open our eyes. No wonder we can't sleep. Even if we manage to drop into bed for the six hours researchers claim most of us spend there, our minds are full of what-ifs, why-did-we's, and what's-on-the-agenda-tomorrows.

This type of rumination and agitation ignites stress hormones that keep us in a state of perpetual arousal. So even if we *do* manage to fall asleep, chances are we'll wake later, wake early, or not be able to reach the deeper levels of restorative sleep we need.

That's why most of us should make a serious attempt to simplify our lives, says Cecile Andrews, Ph.D., a pioneer in simple living and author of *Slow Is Beautiful: New Visions of Community, Leisure, and Joie de Vivre*. Draw up a list of what's important, then draw up a list of what you have to do the next day and compare the two.

What's important to you—the sense of purpose that guides you, the values that you use in making decisions, how you affect the world around you, and whether or not you actually do things you think are important—will slowly become very clear.

"It's really about aligning life with values," adds Rebecca Gould, Ph.D., an associate professor who studies simple-living practices at Middlebury College in Vermont. "There never is a perfect alignment. But to what extent can you bring your life and your values together?" That's the challenge.

The second step is to take a big breath and start crossing things off your to-do list, says Dr. Andrews. It's a bit humbling to realize, but few of us are so unique that there isn't someone else out there who could perform the same tasks just as well.

PUT YOUR JOB IN ITS PLACE. Sleep-stealing on-the-job stress has reached off-the-wall proportions, according to a Canadian health report. And it points a finger at the fact that the workplace no longer has any boundaries. More than half of all employees take work home, 69 percent check their work e-mail from home, 59 percent check voice mail after hours, 30 percent get work-related faxes, and 29 percent keep their cell phones on day and night.

Not surprisingly, 46 percent feel this work-related intrusion is a stressor, and 44 percent report "negative spillover" onto their families.

The problem, however, is not just the fact that work is intruding into familial life, it's also that it's actually interfering with the most effective buffer to workplace stress—the family—as well as active leisure activities, exercise, hobbies, and social activity.

A joint study of 314 workers conducted by the University of South Australia and the University of Rotterdam found that workers with higher levels of these activities were able not only to bounce back from workplace stress better than their always-on-the-job coworkers but also that they slept significantly better.

MANAGE THE ELECTRONICS. This is tough. Few of us can survive for more than 30 minutes without being hooked up to a cell or BlackBerry at the very least. But the technological innovations that were supposed to give us more leisure time have instead made it easier for us to work all the time.

The issue is that by their very nature, they create stress by forcing what Rockefeller University's Bruce McEwen, Ph.D., calls "a wholly artificial sense of urgency" on us. The minute your cell phone rings, you tense. And if your phone rings often, you never get to *un*-tense. That makes it difficult to wind down at night and get to sleep.

The thing is, we don't have to do without our electronics to cut stress. All we have to do is control them. Answer e-mail three times a day instead of every 30 minutes, and turn off the instant notification feature. Moreover, turn off your cell after 6:00 P.M.

THE BLACKBERRY EFFECT

"Having access to information all the time has had a deleterious effect on how much we sleep," says Margaret Moline, Ph.D., former head of the sleep disorders center at Weill Cornell Medical College in White Plains, New York. We haven't yet learned to turn off the stream of information. Like kids with a new Christmas toy, whenever we sit still for five minutes, we whip them out and start browsing online, watching a movie, calling our mothers, adding to the next day's to-do list, paying our bills, or checking our e-mail. In no way, shape, or form is this conducive to sleep.

The bottom line? Turn them off when you come home.

DON'T STAY LATE AT WORK. The prevailing thought is that you have to stay late to get the job done, says Margaret Moline, Ph.D., former head of the sleep disorders center at Weill Cornell Medical College in White Plains, New York. But working right up until bedtime is bound to disrupt your sleep. So go home at a reasonable hour. The truth is that it's better to go home and go to sleep, then come back and do more work in the morning. Studies show that after a good night's sleep, your increased ability to concentrate means that you can work faster—and more accurately.

DON'T CHECK YOUR E-MAIL. At least, not before bed. Researchers at Stanford University have found that the light from your monitor right before bed is enough to reset your whole wake/sleep cycle—and postpone the onset of sleepiness by three hours.

Why These Strategies Work

All the tips in this chapter are intended to help you win what researcher Cliff Saper, M.D., Ph.D., and head of neurology at Harvard Medical School, calls "an arm-wrestling match for your consciousness."

It takes place between two systems in your brain—one designed to keep you awake, the other designed to let you sleep.

One combatant in this match is a group of specialized nerve cells in an area of the brain with the mind-bending name of ventrolateral preoptic nucleus—or VLPO, as scientists call it. The VLPO's nerve cells act as a master switch that turns off the other combatant—the brain's arousal system, which is designed to keep you awake—and lets you sleep.

At the moment your body's internal clock—or the dog having to pee—wakes you in the morning, your internal pressure to sleep is at a minimum. The pressure builds throughout the day, but other cues—light, temperature, and food, for example—signal your body's internal clock to send messages to the VLPO about what's going on in the outer world. Those messages say, "Now is *not* the time for sleep," so you stay alert.

Once you get near your habitual bedtime, however, cues from the external world—the fact that it gets dark, the fact that your internal body temperature drops—signal your internal clock to let the VLPO know it's time to wind down.

The system designed to keep you awake and the one designed to let you sleep wrestle a bit to see whether you stay alert or go to sleep. But the match is actually decided pretty quickly, which is why we frequently refer to the shift into sleep as "dropping off" or "falling" asleep, says Dr. Saper.

"In a match like this, where the two sides can turn each other off, as soon as one side gets a little bit of an upper hand over the other, the other side collapses very easily. The VLPO neurons start firing, and as they do, they turn off the arousal system neurons in the brain so you get sleepy."

What happens in insomnia, adds Dr. Saper, is that the brain is hyperaroused—typically because you're ruminating about something that's emotionally agitating. "If you look at the circuitry in the brain during stress-induced insomnia, the VLPO is trying very hard to turn off arousal," he explains. "But it can't quite do it, because the part of the brain that controls emotion is working equally hard to rev things up. So you enter this weird in-between state where even though you look like you're asleep to an outside observer, you feel as though you spent the whole night awake." And, actually, judging by all the activity in your cerebral cortex, at least part of you did.

So how can someone with insomnia get to sleep and stay asleep?

Sleep clinicians will usually recommend cognitive behavioral strategies that prevent your brain from getting into that ruminative state right before bed to begin with, says Dr. Saper. They will also suggest strategies related to timing, temperature, light/dark exposure, and the like so that you can manipulate your body's internal clock into giving your brain the right cues at the right time for your brain to "fall" asleep. They may also prescribe various sleep medications that will knock you out for at least part of the night.

"Most people who follow all of these strategies will do reasonably well in terms of being able to go to sleep," says Dr. Saper.

Center Yourself

Take time to get in touch with yourself, your feelings, your dreams, and the way you want to live a good, healthy life.

ADMIT THE IMPORTANCE OF SLEEP. Sometimes it seems as though our culture has begun to view the need for sleep as a sign of weakness. It's the new macho—and women are buying into it big-time.

But your body was genetically programmed to spend one-third of its life asleep and to sleep in specific cycles of light sleep, deep sleep, and active-brain sleep. Each cycle takes 90 minutes, and each has a specific assignment that affects thinking, memory, growth, your immune system, and even your weight. Trying to tuck anything that important into an hour here and an hour there just won't get the job done.

BEGIN THE DAY IN GRATITUDE. Take 10 minutes every morning to sit down, close your eyes, and give thanks for every one of the blessings in your life. Name each one and hold it in your thoughts. The sense of gratitude you'll experience will set a serene tone for the entire day—and reduce a day's worth of stress hormones that can trigger insomnia that night.

STRIKE A BALANCE. Toning down a tightly wired nervous system will encourage a balanced sleep/wake cycle, says Dr. Yan-Go. Think about tai chi, meditation, prayer, biofeedback, yoga—any daily activity that allows you to cultivate a peaceful center and a sense of balance.

PLAY WITH FRIENDS. Studies at UCLA reveal that women who have healthy friendships and interactive relationships with their children actually sleep better. The "tend-and-befriend studies," as they are called, conducted by UCLA researcher Shelly Taylor, Ph.D., indicate that when women are stressed, they tend to their children and seek out other women, possibly an ancient survival mechanism that allowed women to band together to protect themselves and their families. The studies show that when this happens, a woman's level of a biochemical called oxytocin, which blocks cortisol, the body's chief stress chemical, is increased, allowing them to rest easier than their wired male counterparts.

USE GUIDED IMAGERY. "Mind/body stuff really works in helping you get to sleep," says Cleveland therapist Belleruth Naparstek, M.S. The imagery seduces the brain into seeing and thinking about other things, while the voice tone, pacing, music, and images will persuade the ramped-up part of your nervous system that it's time to calm down. The imagery will shut down the adrenalin that's keeping you too aroused to sleep, and shoot some calming hormones into your nervous system.

Slip a CD of guided imagery into your CD player, snuggle into bed, turn out the lights, and follow the imagery into sleep. Go to sleep.rd.com for more information.

INVOKE THE RELAXATION RESPONSE. Okay, so it sounds kind of boring. Maybe even useless. But the fact remains that one study after another has demonstrated that progressive muscle relaxation and meditation will block the chemical effects of stress, anxiety, and 24/7 living on your brain—even rebalance your neurochemistry. And practiced right before bed, that often means a night of deep, restorative sleep. Here's the 4-step method pioneered by Herbert Benson, M.D., a cardiologist who heads the Mind/Body Medical Institute in Boston.

1. Choose a word that has deep personal meaning for you such as "peace."

2. Close your eyes and focus your attention on the word. Repeat it silently to yourself. When your attention wanders, as it will, gently bring it back to the word.

3. Take a deep breath and exhale. Begin to consciously relax each of your muscles from your face to your toes.

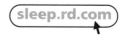

4. When you're finished, continue to focus on your chosen word for another 10 to 15 minutes.

Then allow yourself to gently move into sleep.

"*I visualize myself taking a hot-air balloon ride in the dark. It's incredibly soothing to feel like you're floating above the Earth, looking down on the few lights below, and just drifting. It relaxes me, and I nod off. And I say this as someone who's afraid of heights!*"

—DENISE FOLEY

FIGHT BRAIN CLUTTER. Every time you start thinking about bills or work or kids gone astray, turn your brain off and focus on something that is less stimulating, says sleep researcher Dr. Moline. One woman prays. Another meditates. A third dreams of what she's going to plant in her garden next spring. As long as it doesn't make you worry, you'll be asleep in no time.

Take Your Meds

If you have a health condition that interferes with your regular sleep pattern, work with your doctor to treat it.

THINK ABOUT ORAL CONTRACEPTIVES. Women who use oral contraceptives report less cycle-related insomnia, says Kathryn Lee, Ph.D., a sleep researcher at the University of California at San Francisco. If you're not taking them and premenstrual insomnia is a regular problem, check with your doctor about the possibility of using them.

OR NOT. If you're already using oral contraceptives but you never seem to feel fully rested in the morning, consult with your doctor about an alternative form of birth control. Women who take oral contraceptives have less slow-wave sleep—the deep, restorative sleep that makes you wake up feeling refreshed.

DEAL WITH SLEEP SABOTEURS. Pain, allergies, breathing difficulties, premenstrual hormone warp, shift work, cancer, depression, aging parents, kids—there are a thousand things that can interfere with sleep. We've included some of the most common ones in Part III of this book. Flip through it and see if any pertain to you. If they do, check with your doctor, then follow the experts' tips to get yourself a good night's sleep.

TAME TWITCHY LEGS. If your sleep has been disrupted by twitchy, tingly legs or that creepy-crawly feeling, check with your doctor to see if you have restless legs syndrome or RLS (see page 184). Women who have heavy periods or a genetic predisposition to RLS may need increased amounts of iron and folate, says Dr. Lee. Simple blood tests will help your doctor figure out how much is right for you.

KNOCK YOURSELF OUT. "Sleep meds tend to be most helpful in people with short-term problems," says Lawrence J. Epstein, M.D., past

SNOOZE TO LOSE

An amazing study of 68,000 women conducted at Harvard Medical School reveals that women who sleep five hours a night are 32 percent more likely to gain 30 pounds or more as they get older than women who sleep seven hours or more.

Common sense says that someone who's awake and running around should be using up more calories than someone who's in bed. Running around should make them skinnier, right? But the study, conducted over a 16-year period, reveals that even when the women who slept longer ate more, they still gained less than women who slept less.

president of the American Academy of Sleep Medicine and author of *The Harvard Medical School Guide to a Good Night's Sleep*. "They're that team player who can get you out of trouble in a crunch and prevent a long-term problem. They're for people who want a quick fix rather than a true fix." And to be effective, they still need to be coupled with other good-sleep strategies, such as getting up at the same time every morning.

DOES ONLINE SLEEP THERAPY WORK?

You can bet your Yves Delorme sheets it does.

What's more, it's cheaper, more private, more convenient, and available when *you* have the time—not when a therapist 10 miles away can give you an appointment.

In a study at the University of Uppsala in Sweden, researchers recruited 81 people online to participate in a five-week program of cognitive behavioral therapy (CBT). CBT—which involves learning about what keeps you from sleeping and manipulating your behavior to counteract it in a structured way—is arguably the most effective approach to insomnia. It's as effective as a sleeping pill in the short term and substantially more effective in the long term.

But there are few certified CBT psychologists outside of large cities, and even the four to eight sessions it usually takes to overcome sleep issues doesn't come cheap.

Hence, the interest in whether or not an online CBT would work.

Of those who volunteered online for the study, 57 percent were under age 50, 32 percent were between the ages of 50 and 59, and 9 percent were over age 60—a clear indication that it's not just twentysomethings who are comfortable navigating the online environment, but women of all ages. Volunteers who had sleep apnea, depression, anxiety, and pain were excluded from the study.

Eat, Drink, and Have Cookies
(Low Fat, of Course!)

What you take into your body can seriously affect your sleep patterns—both positively and negatively.

Each study participant maintained a sleep diary two weeks prior to the five-week program, during the program, and for two weeks after its conclusion. For five weeks they received information about what helps sleep and suggestions for specific behaviors, such as how much time they should stay in bed based upon their particular sleep diary.

The result?

Modest but important. By the end of the program, those who had participated went to sleep 29 percent faster, reduced their middle-of-the-night waking by 38 percent, reduced their early-morning awakening by 35 percent, added half an hour to their total sleep time, and increased the quality of their sleep by nearly one-third.

"I believe that Internet CBT can be effective for anyone," says sleep researcher Celyne H. Bastien, Ph.D., a professor of psychology at the Université of Laval in Quebec, who has studied different ways of presenting CBT to those with insomnia. So is CBT via phone. So is CBT in group therapy. So is CBT in individual therapy. Since CBT produces sleep deprivation at first, those who experience insomnia along with another medical condition, such as depression, should use an online program only with their doctor's supervision.

For an online CBT program for insomnia that was developed at the Harvard Medical School, go to www.cbtforinsomnia.com. It will cost you $19.95—about the same as a week's supply of sleeping pills.

DRINK WATER. Or juice. Or decaffeinated diet soda. Drink anything but coffee, hot chocolate, or tea within 6 to 10 hours of bed. Caffeine blocks the effects of adenosine, a chemical produced by your brain that makes you sleepy. In fact, studies have shown that the caffeine in even one cup will rev your circuits enough to reduce both the length and restorative depths of sleep. It will also wake you during the night to urinate.

RESIGN FROM SISTERS WHO SIP. Even if you're a charter member of Divas Uncorked or Sisters Who Sip, you really need to limit alcohol to an afternoon libation, not an after-dinner or before-bed nightcap. Despite its reputation, alcohol sipped at these later times keeps you in the lighter, less restorative stages of sleep in which you're likely to wake if the dog so much as turns over in his bed.

THINK RICE AT 6:00 P.M. Although a well-balanced diet throughout the day is necessary to produce the neurochemicals your brain needs to function efficiently, researchers conducting a study at the University of Sydney in New South Wales discovered that eating a high-carbohydrate meal four hours before bed—jasmine rice, in this case—can cut the time it takes to fall asleep in half.

PUT A LOW-FAT COOKIE AND SOME MILK ON YOUR NIGHTSTAND. The tryptophan in milk will help you feel sleepy, but you need some carbs to get it where you want it to go in your brain, says Mary Susan Esther, M.D., and president of the American Academy of Sleep Medicine. Cookies are her carb of choice. As for tryptophan supplements, she adds, the FDA doesn't recommend them and neither does she. There are still unresolved questions about their safety.

See an Expert

Sometimes you need to discuss your problems with a professional who can recognize your symptoms and offer guidance.

TALK TO A SLEEP DOC. If you suspect you have a sleep disorder involving breathing difficulties, restless legs, or narcolepsy, ask your primary-care physician for a referral to a sleep center for testing, diagnosis, and treatment. If your doctor doesn't know of one in the vicinity, flip to page 214. Chances are, we do.

RETRAIN YOUR BRAIN. The most successful treatment for insomnia is arguably cognitive behavioral therapy. In more than 21 studies involving 470 patients with insomnia from a variety of causes, cognitive behavioral therapy worked just as well as sleeping pills at increasing sleep and improving sleep quality—and it was actually *better* than sleeping pills at helping study participants get to sleep faster.

Despite its intimidating name, cognitive behavioral therapy—or CBT—is simply learning new information about what keeps you from sleeping (the "cognitive" part), and learning how to manipulate your behavior (the "behavioral" part) so that it doesn't. It generally takes only four or five 30-minute sessions to effect change.

Unfortunately, certified cognitive behavioral therapists are scarce. To find one, visit www.academyofct.org and click on "Find a Certified Cognitive Therapist." Fill in your zip code or city and state on the pop-up, and a list of therapists in your area will appear.

If none do, or if you don't have time for even the small number of sessions CBT requires, you can visit www.cbtforinsomnia.com. (See page 31 for more information.)

LIMIT YOUR TIME IN BED. It sounds absolutely bizarre, but one of the most effective strategies to combat insomnia is to restrict the number of hours you spend in bed.

The reason is that most people who have been struggling with insomnia will do seemingly practical things like go to bed a couple of hours early to try to sleep. It rarely works, researchers have found, so most of us will spend, say, seven hours in bed when we only sleep for five.

But remember what we said in a previous tip: Don't stay in bed when you're awake or the association you make (bed = awake) can program

THE QUICK FIX

Yeah, we know. You didn't sleep well last night. So why not take a nap?

Studies show that not only will you feel better almost immediately, says Sara Mednick, Ph.D., a sleep medicine researcher at the University of California at San Diego and author of *Take a Nap! Change Your Life,* but a daily nap of between 20 and 90 minutes before 4:00 P.M. will also increase your mental performance, reduce your chances of gaining weight, and make you feel a whole lot more like having sex after dinner than you probably do now. What's more, it won't affect your nighttime sleep.

All told, a nap, according to Dr. Mednick, will:

- Increase your on-the-job alertness by 100 percent

- Sharpen your thinking so you make more accurate judgments and better decisions

- Ramp up your productivity

- Regenerate skin cells so you look younger

- Increase your sex drive

- Help you lose weight by altering metabolism and shifting chemicals that affect appetite

- Reduce your risk of heart attack, stroke, irregular heartbeat, high blood pressure, and other cardiovascular problems

- Lift your mood by bathing your brain in the neurotransmitter serotonin

- Speed up your ability to perform motor tasks, like typing, operating machinery, even swimming

- Improve your accuracy—in everything

- Improve the way your body processes carbs, which reduces your risk of diabetes

- Sharpen your senses so you take in what's important in your environment—and screen out the 24-hour culture chatter that surrounds us

- Put your brain into its creative gear so you can come up with fresh ideas

- Trigger a naturally occurring hormone that blocks the destructive chemicals produced by stress

- Boost your ability to learn something new—and, better yet, remember it

- Zap the need for drugs like caffeine and alcohol to manipulate your mood and energy level

- Relieve migraines

- Improve your nighttime sleep by eliminating that wired feeling and thus shutting off the brain chatter

- Make you feel good all over

you for insomnia. That's one of the reasons why limiting your time in bed is important. Another is that you're increasing the pressure on your brain to sleep.

To see how much you're really sleeping, sleep medicine specialists advise that you keep a sleep diary for a couple of weeks. Write down when you go to bed, when you wake up, and how many hours you actually sleep.

Once you have a sense of the number of hours you actually sleep, stay in bed for only that number. If you find that you're sleeping only six hours a night even though you're in bed for eight, go to bed at your usual time and set your alarm clock for six hours later.

The first couple of days will be tough. You might not fall asleep right away, so you could end up more sleep deprived than you are now. So avoid driving, operating any kind of machinery, drinking, making important decisions, talking to your mother-in-law, fighting with your partner, and picking up small children.

If, at the end of a week, you're sleeping the full six hours for six out of seven nights, you can increase your time in bed by 15 or 20 minutes. If you're sleeping less than six hours for six out of seven nights, subtract 15 or 20 minutes from your time in bed.

Two caveats:

- One, this technique should be done under the care of a sleep medicine specialist—particularly if you're depressed or taking any medication. Sleep deprivation under these circumstances can be dangerous. It can make depression worse. Moreover, the end-of-the-week adjustments sound simple, but they really should be made by someone who knows the chemical effects of sleep—and the lack thereof—on the brain. If you try to do it yourself, you could get into deep space before you know you're there.

- Two, under no circumstances should you ever allow yourself less than five hours a night in bed. The resulting drowsiness could make you a danger to yourself or others—particularly if you get behind the wheel.

Change Your Ways

You might be surprised to find out just how significant these simple suggestions prove to be. Give them a chance to improve your sleep—and your life.

JOIN THE POD PEOPLE. Want to get some sleep *and* boost job performance by 34 percent?

"Take a 26-minute nap," says Sara Mednick, Ph.D., research scientist at the University of California at San Diego and author of *Take a Nap! Change Your Life.* Studies show that one nap of up to 90 minutes between the hours of 1:00 and 4:00 P.M. will reduce your sleep debt, invigorate your day, boost your job performance, and not affect night sleep, says Dr. Mednick.

"To start, lie down at the same time every day for 20 minutes without the expectation of falling asleep," she says. "That way, you're teaching your body that it's okay to relax in the middle of the day." Eventually your body will believe you, and you'll doze off. Set your watch or cell phone to wake you up—and feel free to expand the time to sleep.

Finding a place to sleep can be tricky. Your car is one place, outside under a tree in a crime-free park is another. Or if you're in a large city, check out the sleep pods some businesses rent out specifically for naps.

But what about your job? "If you can a take 20-minute break to run to Starbucks for coffee," says Dr. Mednick, "you can find 20 minutes for a nap."

If your employer is dubious about the idea, send them to Dr. Mednick. She'll show him or her the NASA studies demonstrating that napping gives us a mental edge.

WORK IT. "Exercise improves sleep as effectively as benzodiazepines in some studies," reports Kalyanakrishnan Ramakrishnan, M.D., an associate professor at the University of Oklahoma Health Sciences Center. On average it reduces the time it takes to get to sleep by 12 minutes, and it increases total sleep time by 42 minutes. And it doesn't take much. Studies at the University of Arizona show that walking six blocks at a normal pace during the day significantly improves sleep at night for women. Scientists suspect that exercise sets your biological clock into a consistent wake/sleep pattern, or it may boost the brain's production of serotonin, a neurochemical that encourages sleep.

Just make sure you finish your walk at least two hours before bed. Any later and the energizing effect of the activity can actually keep you up.

KEEP A WORRY BOOK. "Put a 'worry book' beside your bed," suggests UCLA's Dr. Yan-Go. When you wake and start worrying, jot down everything you're worrying about and any strategies you've thought of that will solve the problems to which they're related. Then close the book, put it on your nightstand, turn out the light, and go back to sleep. Your worries will be waiting for you in the morning.

> "For some reason 2:00 A.M. is when the worried mind awakens and starts zapping you with all the things you've either forgotten to do or might forget to do. Just the mere act of jotting down these things can unburden the mind and wake you up enough out of the worry zone to go back to sleep. The fact that often you can't read your middle-of-the-night scrawls the next morning is beside the point."
> —LAURA KELLY

FORGET ANDERSON. Given the fact that most late-night newscasts tend to feature murder, mayhem, and man's inhumanity to man, these are bound to turn on every arousal mechanism your body owns. No way are you going to drift into a peaceful sleep after 30 to 60 minutes of watching violence and disturbing stories. So ditch the late news. Watch it in the morning when that shot of adrenalin it triggers will help you fight rush-hour traffic.

FORGET STEPHEN. Stephen King thrillers and every other scary book are absolutely verboten if you expect to sleep, says Becky Wang-Cheng, M.D., a medical director at Kettering Medical Center in Ohio. No one sleeps when they're expecting something from under the bed to grab them. Kids aren't the only ones afraid of monsters.

FORGET HOWARD. Like to catch the foul ball's late-night reruns on satellite radio? Keep the Shock Jock on morning-drive time. For some people it's hard to sleep after that much—um—"stimulation."

HAVE SEX INSTEAD. Enjoy a quickie, suggests Dr. Wang-Cheng. Some 44 percent of midlife women say they don't have time for sex. But the Big O is still one of the most sleep-inducing agents around. Just don't forget to protect yourself against an unanticipated side effect that could appear nine months later. Now that would *really* trash your sleep!

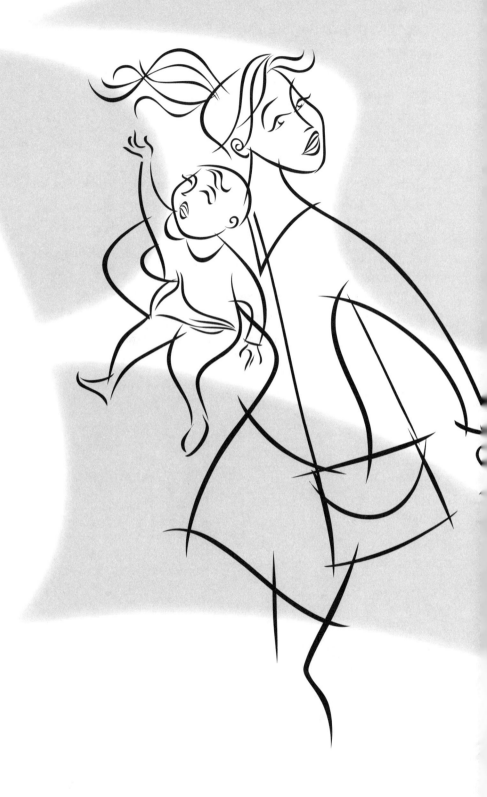

Part III

Sleep Saboteurs
across the
Life Span

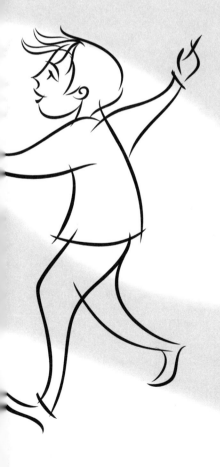

Family Stressors

Women build strong families. We do it by nurturing children, partners, parents, dogs, hamsters, and just about anyone else who wanders in the front door. But there *is* a price.

- 74 percent of stay-at-home moms report they have insomnia almost every night, according to a poll by the National Sleep Foundation. A stunning 39 percent also say they are too tired for sex.
- 72 percent of working moms with school-age children have insomnia.
- 46 percent of working married women with either grown children or no children report they don't get enough sleep—and 38 percent are too tired for sex.

> **44 percent** of working moms report they're **too tired for sex.**

So what's keeping us awake? Dogs, jobs, and health are certainly factors. So are the people we love: Kids. Restless bed partners. Aging parents.

Here's how to love them and *still* get a good night's sleep!

Kids

Moms don't sleep. Not during pregnancy. Not after the kids are born. Not after they're in school. And especially not after they start driving. In fact, a totally unscientific poll of mothers recently revealed that no mom sleeps until her kids are grown and out of the house.

Part of the reason is that we're good parents. We try to give our kids a clean home, clean clothes, and a modicum of attention.

One Woman's Story

MARTHA MURRAY: Sleepless in Fort Myers

There's just one reason why Martha Murray, a Fort Myers, Florida, home-maker, can't sleep, and its name is Sara.

Sara has just turned 16, gotten her driver's license, fallen in love, and uploaded a page on MySpace.

Martha, who had made her daughter watch the *Dateline* series "To Catch a Predator," was very dismayed. "We told her we didn't want her on MySpace. We had her read newspaper stories about girls being lured by predators. We thought we had gotten through to her. Then a friend of mine told us, `Your daughter has a MySpace page.' "

Martha shakes her head. "When your children are babies, you don't get enough sleep because they're awake at all hours. When they're teenagers, you don't sleep because they make you worry."

Teenagers are actually a worry-generating industry. Aside from MySpace, Martha worries about her daughter's driving skills, other drivers on the road, whether or not her daughter is speeding, who's in the car with her, and whether or not she's really going where she says she is.

In the hour before bedtime, 60 percent of us are still doing household chores, reveals a poll by the National Sleep Foundation, while 37 percent of us are doing things with our kids.

A second reason that we're not sleeping is that sometimes our kids are too wired to settle into sleep right away or perhaps it's because they just haven't learned how to get to sleep independently.

A third is that every once in a while, all kids have sleeping problems at night—nightmares, illness, wet beds, just to name a few. Unfortunately, for whatever reason, 47 percent of us have to handle

And she may have cause: Little sister Megan has already told Martha that sister Sara drives too fast, and a neighbor recently told Martha that she saw Sara talking on a cell phone as she drove—a safety no-no of which Sara is very aware.

"From day one we talked to Sara about how the car is like a weapon and you have to be aware of how everyone else around you is driving," says Martha.

But those conversations seem to have gone in one teenage ear and out the other. As a result, Martha worries whenever Sara's out with the car, whether she's simply driving to and from school for a basketball game or over to a friend's house to study. In fact, Martha's biggest sleep problem is the fact that she can't fall asleep until she hears her daughter come home.

It's not that she tries to stay awake; Martha says she just can't sleep until she knows Sara is home safely.

In any case, Martha expects to be sleeping better for the next month. A few days ago she discovered that Sara had lied to her about where she was going and with whom. So she yanked Sara's driving privileges for the next 30 days.

True, she'll have to go back to chauffeuring Sara around. But at least she'll be well rested. For a while.

24 percent of married women have given up sex—whether it's because we're so exhausted we prefer sleep or because we're so irritated at our partner is anybody's guess.

those challenges alone. Whether it's because of divorce, disinterest, or poor parenting, there's no one else there but us to get up in the middle of the night to cuddle a miserable, frightened child.

But we're not the only ones who are losing sleep. So are our kids. Studies show that 40 percent of children report they don't get enough sleep. And at least one survey reveals that 20 percent of teens fall asleep in school on a regular basis.

TAKE TECHNOLOGY
OUT OF THE BEDROOM

Electronics are sleep stealers, says Jodi Mindell, Ph.D., associate director of the Sleep Center at the Children's Hospital of Philadelphia. A whopping 40 percent of school-age children and 20 percent of preschoolers have TVs in the bedroom. "Get them out," says Dr. Mindell. "And take out the computers, Game Boys, and cell phones as well."

A recent study in Germany of 11 healthy boys ages 12 to 14 revealed that when the boys played an interactive computer game called *Need for Speed* for 60 minutes or watched an exciting DVD, such as a *Harry Potter* or *Star Trek* movie, two to three hours before bed, the heart-pounding action-adventure stories and games seriously affected their sleep. The boys took longer to fall asleep and spent less time in the stage of deep restorative sleep— the kind necessary to build strong bodies and sharp minds.

How Much Sleep Do Kids Need?

Age	Amount of Sleep (hours)
1–3	12–14, including naps
3–5	11–13, including naps
5–12	10–11
13–19	9–10

Source: The National Sleep Foundation.

What's more, a study of 1,656 schoolchildren between the ages of 13 and 16 revealed that 62 percent of them use their cell phones after they've gone to bed. The researchers followed the kids for a year and found that those who used their cell phones after bedtime less than once a week doubled the chance they would feel tired the next day.

Those who used their cell phone after bedtime once a week tripled the chance they would feel tired—while those who used their cell phone more than once a week after bedtime were a whopping *five* times more likely to be very tired than their friends who did not.

The researchers also took a look at precisely when the teens were calling each other after they were supposed to be asleep. Use of the cell right after bedtime doubled the odds of being very tired the next day. Using it between midnight and 3:00 A.M. increased the odds by nearly 400 percent.

Help for Sleepless Moms

Here's how to get the housework done, give your children the attention they need, and help your kids get the sleep they need—so *you* can, too. (For more tips for new moms, see "Your New Baby Sleep Strategy," on page 134.)

LOWER YOUR EXPECTATIONS. "I think a lot of us are type-A working moms," says Jodi Mindell, Ph.D., associate director of the Sleep Center at the Children's Hospital of Philadelphia and author of *Sleep Deprived No More: From Pregnancy to Early Motherhood.* "We put a lot of pressure on ourselves. We think we need to be the perfect mom and never lose patience with our kids. We think we need to make sure the house always looks good and that we need to serve gourmet meals when people would be just as happy with spaghetti and meatballs." But you don't have to be the perfect parent, says Dr. Mindell. "Lower your expectations. You don't have to be the perfect gourmet cook or have every holiday decoration. You don't have to be the best housekeeper. You need balance—and part of that balance is in knowing that pizza with veggies or hot dogs with baked beans is fine."

HAVE YOUNGER CHILDREN SLEEP INDEPENDENTLY. Sleeping with younger kids or lying down with them as they fall asleep is fine, says Dr. Mindell. But the problem is, if you lie down with your 3-year-old at bedtime, when she wakes up in the middle of the night, she's going to need you to lie down with her again before she can fall back asleep. So if you want to keep your own sleep from being disrupted, you need to help her understand that she can get back to sleep on her own.

There are many ways to help a child sleep independently, adds Dr. Mindell. One is the sleeping-bag trick. If your child wants to sleep with you, just put a sleeping bag on the floor and tell your child that that's where he or she can stay. Then, night after night, gradually move the sleeping bag away from your bed toward the bedroom door, and then eventually down the hall to his or her own room. It can take a while, but sooner or later the child will gain the confidence to sleep independently. In the end everybody sleeps—and you may even regain your sex life.

GET TODDLERS AND PRESCHOOLERS TO BED BY 7:30 P.M. That gives them 30 minutes to fall asleep and a good 11 hours of sleep time. That, along with a nap or two, is all they need. And if you stick to that schedule, it will give you a few moments to unwind before bed yourself.

GET PRETEENS TO BED BY 8:30 P.M. That gives them 30 minutes to fall asleep and 10 hours to sleep by the time they have to get up at 7:00 A.M. If they need to get up earlier, they should go to bed earlier as well.

GET TEENS TO BED BY 9:00 P.M. Or so. Yeah, it's a challenge. And they're not just being difficult when they say, "But, Mom, I'm not sleepy!" Starting at puberty, the body's biological clock shifts by about two hours. So although your 13-year-old may be able to go to bed at 9:00 P.M. and fall asleep, your 15-year-old probably can't fall asleep until 11:00 P.M.

Unfortunately, this—what scientists call delayed sleep phase—is why most teens seem sleepy all the time. And combined with the fact that the switch from middle school to high school during those years usually means they have to get to school even earlier than ever clearly spells out a recipe for trouble, says Dr. Mindell.

A whopping 20 percent of teens report they fall asleep in school, and studies have found that teens who do not get enough sleep (see table on page 47) are at an increased risk for depression, rage, use of stimulants and alcohol, low grades, and automobile accidents. A study in North Carolina found, for example, that sleepy drivers under the age of 25 were responsible for more than 25 percent of all fall-asleep crashes in that state.

Some enlightened schools are beginning to talk about starting the school day later so teens have a better chance of getting adequate sleep. Another way to handle the issue, says Dr. Mindell, is to use light therapy. Light enters the eyes, shoots down the optic nerve to the brain, tinkers with brain chemicals, and resets the body's biological clock. To get that process started, simply expose your teen to as much sunlight as possible.

Have them eat breakfast in a sunny part of the home, keep blinds and drapes open to allow as much sun into the home as possible, and don't let your kids wear sunglasses to school. All this light will help reset their biological clock and help them fall asleep at an earlier hour.

ESTABLISH BEDTIME ROUTINES. Kids should always do three or four calming activities before bed, says Dr. Mindell, and they should be exactly the same activities every night. Bath, reading, prayer—whatever you choose, its daily repetition literally cues your child's body that it's time to sleep. One note: A National Sleep Foundation poll indicates that reading as a part of the bedtime routine is associated with kids falling asleep faster and sleeping better. And don't forget your teen, adds Dr. Mindell. A routine is just as important for a 15-year-old as it is for a toddler.

GET THE KIDS TO HELP WITH HOUSEWORK. Start when they're eight or nine. Do the dishes together, fold laundry together, count socks. Hand them a dust mop or broom. It frees you so that you can unwind in the hour before bed and thus sleep better. Tell your kids exactly that. It will send them the clear message that sleep is important.

GET TO BED BY 11:00 P.M. Let the dust bunnies go. Forget any laundry left on the floor. Start to practice your own bedtime routine at 10:00 P.M. and slip between the sheets at 11:00 P.M. You may feel so good the next morning that you'll work with the kids to get yourself into bed even earlier. Maybe your bed partner will even lend a hand. And who knows? Maybe you'll have the energy to make love to him in the morning.

Restless Bed Partners

Okay, let's face it: If your bed partner's not sleeping, you aren't, either. Yet a whopping 76 percent of us are sleeping with a restless spouse, according to a National Sleep Foundation poll—and nearly half of them wake in the middle of the night or at the crack of dawn on a regular basis.

It's sad that so many of our partners are tossing and turning, but what it's doing to us is equally tragic. A look at the stats confirms this:

- 55 percent of us have developed insomnia.
- 78 percent of us have developed a sleep disorder.
- 30 percent of us practically fall asleep at our desks three days a week.

> "I didn't have a sleep problem until I got married. My husband just never stopped tossing and turning all night. I wasn't getting any quality sleep at all. I didn't want to start off my marriage in separate bedrooms, so I talked him into going to a sleep center."—JENNIE THORNTON

- 28 percent of us have missed a day of work or some event in the past three months because of our partner's keeping us up.
- Our risk of sleep apnea has increased by 27 percent.
- It takes us nearly *twice* as long to fall asleep as it does our friends who have partners who sleep.
- Only 26 percent of us get a good night's sleep even a *few* nights each month.
- 35 percent of us have developed relationship problems with our partner because of his sleep disorder.

Think that's a bit extreme? A study conducted some years ago at the Mayo Clinic revealed that a snoring partner wakes his non-snoring partner an average of *20 times a night*—with an average sleep loss of one solid hour a day.

A New Mattress Can Heat Up Your Sex Life

A 2007 poll by the Better Sleep Council reveals that the secret to a healthy relationship may be hiding—uh—"under your sheets."

When asked how a new mattress affected their relationship with a bed partner, here's what respondents replied:

- 52 percent felt more cordial to one another during the day.

- 40 percent experienced less sleep disruption from their partner's tossing and turning—and felt less annoyed.

- 27 percent felt they wanted to spend more time in bed with their partner.

- 26 percent reported that their sex life heated up significantly.

Makes you wonder if there's a correlation between insomnia and divorce, doesn't it?

But snoring isn't the only thing that may be keeping your partner up. It could be anything from the bedroom temperature to a medication he's taking, a hard day at the office, or even unresolved tensions in your relationship, says Donna Arand, Ph.D., clinical director of the Sleep Disorders Center at Kettering Hospital in Dayton, Ohio.

The latter is particularly destructive—to sleep as well as the relationship—and you should try to figure out whether specific subjects are triggering either arguments or those tight-lipped, I'm-keeping-my-temper-on-a-leash comments some of us tend to lay on our partners when we're upset.

If there are specific issues, simply resolving not to talk about them after dinner will help your sleep immeasurably, says Dr. Arand.

If there aren't, if there are larger issues that haunt the perimeter of your relationship, then it's time to see a marriage counselor.

Dealing with a Restless Bed Partner

Sleep loss can kill a relationship. In a study at the University of California at Berkeley, researchers found that sleep deprivation fractures brain mechanisms that tame our emotional responses to stressors. In other words, once provoked by a spouse or significant other after sleep deprivation, there's no guarantee we will play nice. And that kills sex and considerably lowers the chances of staying together. Here's how to make sure that doesn't happen.

TALK TO YOUR PARTNER. Be factual, brief, and don't bring in other issues. Avoid personal criticism. Women who refuse to discuss sleep issues with their partners may be putting themselves at risk for more than insomnia. A Maryland study recently found that women who "self-silenced" during conflicts with their spouses were four times more likely to die over a 10-year period than women who did not.

EMPHASIZE THAT IT'S "OUR" PROBLEM. That makes it clear that you're in this for the long haul and you've got his back.

ENCOURAGE HIM TO GET HELP. Suggest he make an appointment with your family doctor to discuss the issue and consider whether or not a referral to a sleep center certified by the American Academy of Sleep Medicine would help.

USE PROPS. Eye masks, ear plugs, white-noise machines, mattresses with "firmness" controls, feather boas—use whatever it takes to increase the likelihood that you'll sleep through your partner's tossing and turning.

SEPARATE. If the problem is long-term, think twin beds or separate rooms. You can always tiptoe in for a morning cuddle after a good night's sleep.

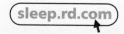

Aging Parents

Watching your elderly mother nod off in front of the television may bring soft smiles of affection from your family—*"Awwww, there goes Grandma again!"* But if they saw your mother up and pacing the floor at 4:00 A.M., they might not think her naps were so endearing. Not only can't *she* sleep, but you can't, either—not when you know she's so miserable.

As our aging parents continue to live longer than any other generation, many of us are increasingly involved in their health and well-being, whether they live with us or not.

One woman is roused from sleep every morning at 4:00 A.M. by the sounds of her 80-year-old mother making oatmeal in the kitchen. By the time she hears the clang of the pot going into the sink to be washed, the sound of the stainless-steel spoon scraping round and round and round the pot as her mother stirs the oatmeal has already raised her blood pressure and driven sleep away.

Another eighty-something woman, who lives on her own, has started calling her niece on the phone in the middle of the night. "I have to get to the hospital!" she demands tearfully. "Your uncle needs me!" Her niece gently reminds the elderly woman that her husband died two years ago, then spends an hour consoling the grief-stricken woman.

With help from geriatric doctors, professional caregivers, and therapists who specialize in the challenges of old age, most of us painstakingly work these issues out.

But as we do, we're torn between the need

A study at Harvard Medical School reveals that bright-light therapy can reduce "sundowning," the agitated behavior that frequently occurs in those with Alzheimer's disease at sundown. The more severe the behavior, the more effective the therapy.

Conditions That Can Disrupt Elders' Sleep

- Alzheimer's disease
- Arthritis
- Asthma
- Cancer
- Chronic obstructive pulmonary disease
- Diabetes
- Enlarged prostate
- Gastroesophageal reflux disease

- Heart disease
- Heartburn
- High blood pressure
- Incontinence
- Osteoporosis
- Parkinson's disease
- Restless legs syndrome
- Sleep apnea
- Stroke

to help and the need to sleep. Eventually, usually in the middle of a dark, restless night, we begin to realize that if *we* want to sleep, we need to help *them* get to sleep as well.

The Myths of Elder Sleep

Until recently, most of us simply assumed that getting old meant nodding off in our chair during the day and sleeping less at night. After all, that's what our aging parents have been complaining about, right?

But scientists have recently begun to question our assumptions about what's keeping our aging parents up. In fact, they're beginning to think that insomnia is not a natural consequence of aging but is actually the result of some very specific problems that have very specific solutions.

The problems seem to fall into four areas, says researcher Sonia Ancoli-Israel, Ph.D., a professor of psychiatry at the University of California at San Diego and a recent president of the Sleep Research Society.

For one thing, "the older we get, the more problems we have with our health," she explains. "Depression, pain from arthritis or from cancer, neurological disorders like Alzheimer's, and organ system failures that are a result of heart disease, pulmonary disease, and kidney failure—all these things will interrupt sleep."

Second, "all the medications we give older adults to treat all these medical and psychiatric illnesses can also interfere with sleep—particularly medications that are stimulating or activating when taken in the evening."

A third cause is the increase in sleep disorders (see page 180) that seems to occur with aging—restless legs syndrome and sleep apnea, in particular—and a fourth is changes in our biological clocks.

"Changes in our body's circadian rhythms make the ability to get the sleep we need more difficult," explains Dr. Ancoli-Israel. "As we get older, our biological rhythm advances such that older people get sleepier earlier in the evening—around 6:00, maybe 7:00 or 8:00 P.M.

MEDS THAT CAN DISRUPT ELDERS' SLEEP

- Antidepressants
- Anti-arrhythmics
- Antihistamines
- Beta-blockers
- Bronchodilators
- Calcium channel blockers
- Clonidine
- Corticosteroids
- Cardiovascular drugs
- Decongestants
- Diuretics
- Gastrointestinal drugs
- Theophylline
- Thyroid hormones

"If they went to bed at that hour, they would sleep their regular amount of time—that is, about seven or eight hours. But do the math: That means that they would wake up at 3, 4, or 5 in the morning, which, of course, is the biggest complaint of older adults: *I'm waking up in the middle of the night, and I can't get back to sleep.*

"The reason that they can't is that their biological clock is waking up," says Dr. Ancoli-Israel. "Their physiological night is over."

In many cases, however, our aging parents are not going to bed at 7:00 or 8:00 P.M., when they first get sleepy. Instead, they try to stay awake until the more acceptable bedtime of 9:00, 10:00, or 11:00 P.M.

What that frequently means, however, is that they sit down after dinner in front of the TV and doze off. "They might sleep for half an hour or hour," says Dr. Ancoli-Israel. "Then they wake up."

She chuckles. "But if you ask them if they nap in the evening, they say no, because sleeping in front of the TV doesn't seem to count."

Unfortunately, once our elders get into bed, they find that they can't sleep. Since they've just slept for an hour, why should they? The chemical pressure to sleep from your biological clock just isn't there. So they toss and turn for hours—then wake up at 4:00 A.M. Their nap time, plus the hours in bed, have equaled a full night's sleep.

One other thing that frequently keeps our elders from a restorative sleep are life stressors. Just because our parents are old, it doesn't mean they don't have as much stress as we do, says Cathy A. Alessi, M.D., a professor at UCLA and associate director of clinical health services research at the Los Angeles Veterans Administration Healthcare System.

They may not be worrying about childcare or a demanding employer, but they *are* facing major stressors, such as retirement, trying to make ends meet on Social Security or a retirement plan crafted in World War II, downsizing into smaller homes, transferring to assisted-living facilities, the loss of friends and partners through illness and death, even their own mortality.

In some ways the things our aging parents have to face are the toughest challenges life will ever demand.

Getting Mom (or Dad) to Sleep

Poor sleep in our elders is caused by very specific problems. Here are some very specific solutions to counter them so *everyone* in the family can get a good night's sleep.

RESET THE CLOCK. Since much of an aging parent's insomnia may be caused by natural changes in their biological clock as they age, you can help them reset that clock simply by doing two things, says sleep researcher Sonia Ancoli-Israel, Ph.D., a professor of psychiatry at the University of California at San Diego.

One, encourage them to get out into the natural sunshine every day, as late in the day as possible. Light will shoot down the optic nerve into the brain, where it will trigger a cascade of brain chemicals that will help them stay awake in the evening. It's a good idea to suggest they leave their sunglasses at home to get the maximum effect. On the other hand, if they go out in the morning, they should be encouraged to wear sunglasses, since morning light can actually aggravate their problem.

Two, suggest they use light therapy, particularly during the winter, when late afternoon light is dim. Get them a light box—a device that generates up to 10,000 lux of light—and suggest they sit near it every evening sometime between 7:00 and 9:00 P.M. They don't need to stare directly at the box but can watch television, read a book, or do any other sedentary activity. If the box emits 10,000 lux, they should sit in front of it for 20 to 30 minutes.

There are two types of light boxes: one that emits blue light and another that emits full-spectrum white light. Although blue light is more effective for younger people, it doesn't penetrate cataracts effectively.

So get them a light box with full-spectrum white light, says Dr. Ancoli-Israel. Check out the list of manufacturers at www.sltbr.org.

CHANGE TIMING OR DOSAGE OF MEDS. Have your elders talk with their doctors about whether any of their medications might be disrupting their sleep. In many cases, says Dr. Ancoli-Israel, changing the timing or dosage of a medication can relieve insomnia. For example, a blood pressure pill taken in the morning that makes them drowsy during the day can often be switched to bedtime. And there it does double duty—it not only lowers their blood pressure but also helps them drift into sleep.

WATCH FOR SLEEP DISORDERS. If your parents complain of "twitchy legs" or disruptive snoring, suggest that they ask their doctors to evaluate them for restless legs syndrome or sleep apnea.

TREAT MEDICAL CONDITIONS. If arthritis pain, for example, is keeping your elders up, suggest they ask for a pain medication. Treating a medical condition can often have the positive aspect of inducing sleep.

GET THEM MOVING. Suggest you go for a walk, go line dancing, or spend an afternoon shopping. A Brazilian study recently found that elderly women who stay active sleep an hour longer each night than those who are sedentary. What's more, they wake up less throughout the night.

PAY ATTENTION TO SLEEP BASICS. Encourage your parents to use the bedroom only for sleeping and keep it dark, quiet, and cool. Suggest they get rid of their bedside clock so they can't watch it all night. They might also want to avoid alcohol after 6:00 P.M., set aside a "worry time" in the early evening, and take a warm bath before bed.

GIVE CRAZY SOCKS FOR GIFTS. "There's a study out of Switzerland that shows that wearing socks to bed helps induce sleep," says Dr. Ancoli-Israel. Turns out that if you can warm your extremities, it helps drop your core body temperature. And that drop signals your body it's time for sleep.

Stress
and Worry

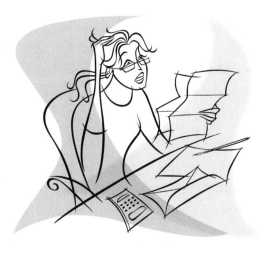

Stress. Its biochemical surge tosses us into a fast-paced hyper-alertness that allows us to dodge an oncoming car, sidestep a fist, or save the data on a crashing computer. But that's in the short term. In the long term, the biochemistry of chronic stress can trigger anxiety and send us spinning toward depression.

A 20-minute nap boosts levels of a natural stress antidote in your brain.

Unfortunately, today's emphasis on a 24/7 workplace, perfect children, a plasma TV in every home, and a size 0—size 0!—waist means that chronic stress is ubiquitous and anxiety a way of life.

And since insomnia is a frequent companion of stress and worry, it also means that probably half the women in your town are pacing the floor at 4:00 A.M. Want some sleep? Kill the stress. Muzzle the anxiety.

Here's how to do it.

Taking Stress to Bed

Turning over for the forty-seventh time that night, 38-year-old Belinda James tried to figure out how she could stretch this week's paycheck to buy food for herself and her two kids, fill up the gas tank, pay the phone bill, have her tooth filled, and pay the rent.

It just wasn't going to happen. She turned over again, punched the pillow a couple of times, and tried to sleep. Instead, a picture of an unfinished report on her desk popped into her mind. If only she'd been able to finish. If only she'd been able to tally that last column of numbers. If only…

Like a lot of women trying to raise a family, hold down a job, and keep life worth living, Belinda James frequently finds herself tossing and turning at 4:00 A.M. as all of her stressors march through her head. There's the ex-husband who expects her to pick up and drop off the kids. The mother who wants her to date. The boss who wants her to increase her output by 20 percent in the next six months. The homeroom teacher who wants to "discuss" her son's behavior. And, of course, the money— for food, phone, gas, dentist, and rent. The list goes on and on.

THE TOP 11 STRESS FOODS

A survey by the American Psychological Association reveals that when you're under stress, you're likely to reach for one of these 11 foods.

1. Chocolate or candy
2. Ice cream
3. Potato chips or tortilla chips
4. Cookies or cake
5. Fast food
6. Pizza
7. Snack crackers
8. Nuts
9. Spreads or dips
10. Fruit
11. Vegetables

Help Me! I'm Up!

When Boston-based naturopathic physician Beth Pimentel can't sleep, it's usually because she's stressed about something that will resolve itself if she just lets it alone.

So instead of ruminating about her stressor when she wakes in the middle of the night, she turns off her mind with a visualization exercise that redirects her attention and induces a state of deep relaxation.

"Resting in bed with the lights off, I place one hand over my lower abdomen and the other over my heart," says Dr. Pimentel. "I try to imagine breathing into my lower hand, expanding my diaphragm, and feeling my belly gently rise with each breath.

"Once I've established a quiet, slow rhythm of breathing, I focus on my heart and the penetrating warmth of my hand. As my awareness settles in my heart, I allow it to expand throughout my chest. Then I allow it to deepen and expand yet again, until my heart has filled my entire body with love.

"Still being aware of my heart, I allow it to expand beyond my body all the way to the edges of the horizon, enveloping and infusing everything it touches with peace, love, and gratitude.

"I rest there for several minutes, in that feeling of spaciousness, and then slowly withdraw my awareness until I am focusing once more on my two hands—one on my abdomen and one on my heart.

"I often fall asleep that way," she adds, "and wake up in the morning with my hands still in place."

Unfortunately, the biochemicals her body generates throughout the day as she tries to deal with these challenges is what keeps her awake at night. "When you're under stress, you get an increase in adrenaline that causes your sympathetic nervous system to go from normal functioning into overdrive," explains Donna Arand, Ph.D., clinical director of the Kettering Hospital Sleep Disorders Center in Dayton, Ohio.

"There's a general overall arousal. Essentially, you're running in fifth gear all the time instead of second."

A Custom Fit

Not everyone responds to stress with insomnia. Heredity, childhood experiences, diet, exercise, personal relationships, and the sheer number of stressors impacting your poor beleaguered body dictate the way you react to stress. In a study conducted at the Finnish Institute of Occupational Health, for example, women who had a pre-existing tendency toward anxiety were twice as likely to develop insomnia than those who did not. Men were even more vulnerable. Men with a preexisting tendency toward anxiety were *three* times more likely to develop insomnia.

"Insomnia is a part of the individual way each of us handles stress," says Dr. Arand. Some people park stress at the bedroom door. Others develop high blood pressure. Still others take it to bed—their minds just won't turn off.

That's not to say that occasional insomnia isn't normal. "Insomnia is a normal response to occasional stress," says Dr. Arand. "If it's the night before your presentation at work or the night before your divorce, it's a natural response."

What's not natural, she explains, is if insomnia becomes chronic. And that usually happens when you focus on the

> **Top 9 Workplace Stressors**
>
> 1. A lack of control over your workload
> 2. No channel of communication to upper management
> 3. The 24-hour workday
> 4. Lack of appreciation
> 5. Inconsistent rewards from management
> 6. Making and discarding goals, plans, or directions without telling the employee why
> 7. Unclear company direction and policies
> 8. Office politics
> 9. Random interruptions
>
> SOURCE: Global Business and Economic Roundtable on Addiction and Mental Health.

One Woman's Story

Whenever Madeline Evans's in-laws come to visit her home in Shaker Heights, Ohio, Madeline's stress level goes through the roof.

"It's not that they aren't good people," she says. "They are. My mother-in-law is vivacious and full of enthusiasm about almost everything—and she's a fun grandmother who loves her grandkids." Her father-in-law is a relaxed kind of guy who longs for peace and quiet, Madeline says. Unfortunately, he doesn't get much—and neither does Madeline whenever her in-laws visit. They constantly bicker with one another, pick fights with others, shout at the dinner table, play games of one-upmanship, and rage at everyone around them over perceived slights.

Adding to the stress, every time Madeline, her husband, Bob, their kids, and her in-laws eat out together, her mother-in-law makes a scene. The elder woman gets snotty and snippy with the wait staff, Madeline reports with a shudder. She always seems to feel the wait staff hasn't treated them properly or served them swiftly enough, and she shows it. Loudly.

"I end up just wanting to disappear, I feel so embarrassed," Madeline says.

To avoid these stressful scenes, Madeline tried cooking at home, but that was worse. "I used to cook big feasts for Bob's family, but no one would ever lift a finger to help with cooking or the cleanup," she says. "They'd just sit around watching TV or yacking while I fumed, too wimpy to ask

fact that you're not sleeping rather than on the stressor that actually caused the problem. You begin to think that insomnia is the problem—and you go to bed expecting to have a problem getting to sleep or staying asleep. As a result, says Dr. Arand, we start thinking, What if it happens again tonight? And, sure enough, it becomes a self-fulfilling prophecy.

for help. And they'd snack all day long, leaving dirty dishes and food scraps all over the place."

The worst thing, however, was when her in-laws would first arrive. "They would arrive with literally a carload of junk they'd picked up, mostly at garage sales," Madeline says. "Old toys, framed pictures, boxes of old books, old clothes, MacDonald's plastic figures. They would dump everything on our living room floor, and then they would insist on showing us each item while exclaiming, 'Isn't this wonderful? Don't you just love this?' "

Madeline and Bob didn't, and when they tried to tell the older couple, it always ended in a screaming match with the older folks saying the younger ones were ungrateful. Madeline knew she had to do something. The stress was making everyone unhappy, and Madeline couldn't sleep.

She settled on a three-part plan and put it into action the next time her in-laws visited. First, she and her husband didn't say a word about the garage sale "finds" dumped in their living room. They let the junk sit, then called the Salvation Army to come and get it when her in-laws left.

Second, Madeline decided to "disappear" several times a day. "I'd just go upstairs to my room and lie down. There was so much noise downstairs," she chuckles, "that no one even noticed I was gone." And third, Madeline ordered takeout for every meal. The family didn't eat out, and Madeline didn't cook. It was perfect.

Madeline laughs. "I find I sleep much better now that I've stopped trying to 'fix' my in-laws' behavior," she says. "They're never going to change. They are who they are."

Supporting the notion that you seemingly have a problem with sleep rather than stress is the fact that you feel so totally rotten the morning after a sleepless night. So you say to your friends at work, "I feel awful. I couldn't sleep a wink last night!" And they all nod their heads knowingly because—guess what?—they didn't sleep so well, either.

So now you've gotten support in blaming the wrong problem. And instead of trying to find a solution to what's actually causing the insomnia—your stressors—you're trying to find ways to catch up with the sleep you missed so you don't feel so darned awful.

"Sleep becomes your overriding thought in life," says Dr. Arand. You start mainlining caffeine during the day, then popping sleeping pills at night. Those strategies may give you a temporary boost in alertness, but in the long run they only exacerbate the problem.

The really insidious thing about this whole mess, says Dr. Arand, is that once you get into this pattern, even when your stressor is eventually eliminated—the rent gets paid, the ex-husband moves out of state, the tooth gets pulled—you've gotten yourself into a pattern of chronic insomnia. So now your problem really isn't stress, it's things like multiple naps erasing the need to sleep at night, too many trips to Starbucks for a caffeine fix, and your expectation that you won't sleep because, of course, you have a "sleep problem."

Fortunately, once you realize what's going on, changing how you handle stress and reestablishing healthy sleep practices will bring back restorative sleep within weeks.

WOMEN'S TOP 10 STRESSORS

Almost half of us lose sleep every month due to one of these 10 stressors, according to the 2007 American Psychological Association Stress Poll.

1. Work
2. Money
3. Workload
4. Children
5. Family responsibilities
6. Your health
7. Family's health
8. Parents' health
9. Housing costs (mortgage or rent)
10. Intimate relationships

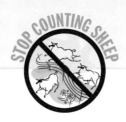

Fixing Stress

When stress interrupts your sleep on a nightly basis, it sets you up for a chronic insomnia that can send you sliding down the rabbit's hole toward sleeping pills, alcohol, and chocolate cake at night and a zillion cups of coffee during the day. Here's how to step back from that precipice.

TARGET THE ENEMY. "Every night a couple of hours before bed, sit down and make a list of all the issues, problems, and things you have to deal with," says Donna Arand, Ph.D., clinical director of Kettering Hospital Sleep Disorders Center in Dayton, Ohio. "Next to each item, write a solution or plan." If you're mad at your mother-in-law, for example, the solution could be to call her and talk it out.

Even if it's not something you want to do, write down your ideas for dealing with each stressor you've listed, urges Dr. Arand. Then mull the solutions over.

When you're ready for bed, put the list by the bedroom door. That way, if thoughts of your problems arise as you're trying to sleep, you can tell yourself, "I've got a plan and I'll work on it tomorrow," says Dr. Arand. The reassuring presence of your plan by the door will give it a concrete reality that will allow you to shift your mind to more peaceful things.

PUT YOUR WORK IN PERSPECTIVE. A Canadian health agency that tracks health-related statistics reported recently that on-the-job stress has reached alarming levels. They point to the fact that the workplace no longer has any boundaries and that work has spread into every corner of your life. It's gotten to the point that 52 percent of employees take work home—almost double the number who did in 1990. What's more, 69 percent of employees check their work e-mail from home, 59 percent check voice mail after hours, 30 percent accept work-related faxes at home, and 29 percent keep their cell phones on at all times.

Not surprisingly, 46 percent feel this work-related intrusion is a stressor, and 44 percent report "negative spillover" onto their families. A poll conducted by the American Psychological Association found that 52 percent of American workers said that work interfered with their responsibilities to their families. The problem, however, is not just that work is intruding into familial life, it's that it's actually interfering with the most effective buffers to workplace stress available.

A joint study of 314 workers conducted by the University of South Australia and the University of Rotterdam found that workers with higher levels of active leisurely activities, such as exercise, hobbies, and social activity, were able not only to bounce back from workplace stress better than their always-on-the-job coworkers but also sleep significantly better than others.

TAKE CHARGE OF YOUR GADGETS. Although each new, more multifaceted electronic device that appears in the marketplace promises to make the logistics of our lives a snap, they may actually tie us into too many never-ending webs. First we have to pay for them. Then we have to master how to use them. Next we have to show them off by contacting our network of business associates and friends. They will, of course, respond in kind.

Being able to keep in touch with the kids is a boon to working parents. Allowing the office to track you down after hours is not. We need to keep the two things separate, save discrete times in the day to receive and answer business e-mails, and learn to screen the after 6:00 P.M. cell phone calls. That goes for the whole rest of the evening as well. It also wouldn't hurt if everyone in the family turned off their devices for a stress-free dinner. And under no circumstances should you check your e-mail right before bed.

DO WITH LESS. According to a poll by the American Psychological Association, 4 of the top 10 stressors we experience are related to money—how we get it and how we spend it. Given that, doesn't it make sense that if we want less and are content with less—smaller houses, fewer gadgets, and simpler forms of transportation—our stress levels will go down?

Perhaps that applies to our career choices as well. Do you really want to work yourself to death to be the woman in charge of the world? Or will just being in charge of a small portion of it make you happy and let you sleep? A recent poll of nearly 2,000 Americans reveals that 22 percent declined a promotion or refused to seek one because they thought the job would be too stressful.

GIVE A NOD TO A NAP. It's doubly unfortunate that stress makes it hard to get to sleep because, chemically speaking, the antidote to stress *is* sleep, says Sara Mednick, Ph.D., a Harvard-trained research scientist at the University of California at San Diego and author of *Take a Nap! Change Your Life*. That's because when you're asleep, your levels of the stress hormone cortisol drop and your levels of growth hormone—cortisol's opposite number—significantly rise.

Unfortunately, if you're getting the typical working woman's six hours of sleep (or less) a night, you're sleep deprived on a chemical level—your cortisol's too high and your growth hormone never gets enough time on the streets to hit its stride.

There is a way to tamp down the cortisol and get a hit of growth hormone during the day, however. And that's by taking a nap.

It's true that several naps during the day, particularly after dinner, will reduce your ability to fall sleep at your usual 11:00 P.M. bedtime, but studies show that one nap of up to 90 minutes between the hours of 1:00 and 4:00 P.M. will not interfere, says Dr. Mednick. In fact, it will reenergize anyone who's not dead.

Begin orienting your body to afternoon naps with a 20-minute period of quiet relaxation that occurs at the same time every day, says Dr. Mednick. If you have a sofa in your office, all the better, but you can create a temporary nap place with a chair and an improvised ottoman. You may want to keep a pillow and an alarm clock at work, too, for nap time. Some cities even have sleeping pod franchises where you can rent a comfortable sleeping chair for 20-minute naps for less than $15.

But what about your job? "If you can take a 20-minute break to run to Starbucks for coffee," says Dr. Mednick, "you can find 20 minutes for a nap." If your employer objects, send him or her to Dr. Mednick. She will be happy to show him data from NASA studies demonstrating that a 26-minute nap boosts on-the-job performance by 34 percent.

RECOGNIZE YOURSELF. How do you deal with stress? Pig out on chocolate mousse? Skip meals? Refill your wineglass a couple of times after dinner? All of these classic stress responses actually make falling asleep and staying asleep more difficult. But if you realize that you're one of those who responds to stress in a way that will sabotage your sleep, plan ahead of time how you're going to handle something you just know is going to raise your stress level.

If you know the big year-end sales conference is coming up next week and you've got some pretty lofty goals to achieve, for example, get into bed an hour early every night *this* week, which will give your body a biochemical boost of stress-proofing growth hormone to ride into the week.

If you know you're going to see your ex when he drops off your daughter Saturday evening, take time out and meditate for 20 minutes before he's supposed to arrive.

Or if you're planning to attend a huge wedding and you know that hanging out with a few hundred people raises your stress level, find a nice quiet spot at the gathering—outdoors under a tree, indoors in an upstairs bathroom, out in your car—where you can take a deep breath, close your eyes for 10 minutes, and enjoy the peace of being alone.

CHECK OUT COMEDY CENTRAL. If you like to unwind in front of the television each evening, tune in to one of the channels that offers a few laughs. Researchers at the University of California at Irvine asked 16 people to watch a funny videotape while the researchers measured various biochemicals related to stress. The result? When study participants watched the tape, their levels of stress hormones dropped significantly and levels of the antistress growth hormone rose 87 percent.

CUT YOURSELF SOME SLACK. If you know a situation will add to your stress level, avoiding it when you're not sleeping may well be the healthiest thing you can do. One woman who worked the counter in a bakery found herself tossing and turning every night as she thought about all her stressors—her kid, the mortgage, her husband's health, the whole nine yards.

But one morning the lack of sleep, her stressors, and the fact that she had to deal with customers niggling back and forth between caraway or sesame seeds put her right on the edge. So she swapped places with a baker in the back of the store. The baker—not unhappy with the change at all—waited on customers while the stressed-out counterwoman peacefully kneaded dough.

That night, the counterwoman slept well.

PLANT AN HERB GARDEN. Line your bedroom windowsill with lavender plants, pinch off some leaves before bed, and slip them into your pillowcase. Studies show that the effects of herbal fragrances such as lavender reduce stress levels. In one study people exposed to lavender showed an increase in the type of brain waves that suggest increased relaxation.

TAKE FIDO TO BED. In one analysis researchers evaluated the heart health of 240 couples, half of whom owned a pet. Those couples with pets had significantly lower heart rates and blood pressure levels when exposed to stressors than the couples who did not have pets—a sign that stress is less likely to be affecting their sleep!

CONNECT. Studies at UCLA reveal that women's friendships and relationships with their children can block stress hormones. Conducted by researcher Shelly Taylor, Ph.D., the "tend and befriend" studies, as they are called, indicate that when women are stressed, they tend to their children and seek out other women. Possibly an ancient survival mechanism that allowed women to band together to protect their children, the studies show that when women tend to their children and hang out with friends, they increase levels of a biochemical called oxytocin, which blocks cortisol, the body's chief stress chemical. The result? Low-stressed women are more likely to sleep at night than their wired male counterparts.

FORGIVE THE PAST. Anger toward someone who has wronged you can trigger a cascade of stress hormones that can haunt you through the night. To prevent that effect, think about how you were hurt, your response, and how you feel right now. Then think about whether or not there's anything in the background of the person who hurt you that explains what he or she did. If there is, put yourself in their shoes—and see if you can't forgive them. If you can, you'll sleep like a baby.

CATCH UP. If you're always running late, sit down with a pencil and paper and see how you're actually allotting your time. Say it takes 40 minutes to get to work. Are you leaving your home on time? You may very well be able to de-stress life a bit just by being realistic. And if you can't find the time for all the activities that are important, maybe you're trying to do too much.

GET PHYSICAL. Burn off a rush of stress with a 15-minute walk. Studies show that those who regularly exercise sleep better than those who don't.

FIND SPIRITUAL FRIENDS. A study conducted by researchers from the University of Washington found that those who routinely hang out with others who share their religious beliefs were less likely to be affected by stress when confronted with major stressors.

DILUTE THE EFFECTS OF STRESSFUL PEOPLE. One example: If you don't get along with your father-in-law but don't want to make an issue of it, invite other in-laws at the same time you invite him. Having other people around will absorb some of the pressure you would normally feel.

DITCH THE MULTITASKING. Can't remember what you did all day or what you accomplished? Boy, that'll jack up your stress level! Unfortunately, multitasking only *looks* as if you're accomplishing a lot. Studies suggest that it actually impairs memory and performance.

Try doing only one thing at a time for a few days. You'll be able to remember what you've accomplished each day and—if you've done a good job—feel relaxed about your work at the end of the day.

TAKE SOME TIME TO SAY THANKS. Take 10 minutes every morning to sit down, close your eyes, and give thanks for the blessings in your life. Name each one, and hold the purpose in your thoughts. The sense of gratitude you'll experience will set a serene tone for the entire day.

CHOOSE NOT TO GET ANGRY. Being angry not only revs your stress motor, it makes you feel bad. So next time someone cuts into your lane on the freeway, recognize your instinctive surge of adrenaline and then decide not to let it control you. Instead, smile and say to yourself, "I'm not going to let someone like that affect how I feel." Amazingly, it works.

COVER THE BASICS. As you work on bringing your stressors under control, pay attention to the basic framework that sleep experts say will set your body's circadian rhythms for nighttime sleep.

"Establish a bedtime routine in which sleep becomes the last step in that routine," adds Dr. Arand. Toss your clothes in the laundry, take a shower, moisturize your body, dry your hair, put on your pj's, slip into bed, and pick up a book. Fifteen minutes later, put it down and turn out the light. "The body loves consistency," says Dr. Arand. "It loves conditioning and rhythm."

Worry

Your mother's not well. Your daughter flunked her biology test. Your husband seems to come home later and later. And your boss seems ticked off about something. So what's not to worry about?

The thing is, most of us have a lot on our plate. But some of us get into a kind of worry jag where we always expect the worse to happen—we're a bit hyper, a bit irritable, we're exhausted a lot of the time, and we just can't sleep.

Of course, who *could* sleep when you just know your mother's probably got a heart condition, your daughter's going to flunk out of school, your husband's tired of looking at you, and you're about to get fired?

See the pattern? Worry, worry, worry. It's a problem that affects some 4 million people in the United States, most of them women.

Unfortunately, some of us are more prone than others to this type of worry jag—technically designated as a generalized anxiety disorder, or GAD, when it lasts for six months or longer. That's because although GAD often seems to start with a buildup of specific stressors—your mother complained of chest pain or your boss dumped 46 years' worth of work on your desk, for example—the fact is that it also seems as though some of us may be hardwired in such a way that we're more likely to respond to stress with the kind of chronic worry that eventually becomes GAD.

Researchers haven't figured all that out just yet, but they have noted a relationship between stress and the development of GAD. In a study at King's College in London, for example, researchers who had followed nearly a thousand men and women from birth took a look at the effects of work stress on study participants when they finally reached the age

> "When I can't sleep because I have too many to do's on my mind, I do a brain 'dump.' I keep a pad and pen on my nightstand and write down the to do list to get it off my mind and transferred to a piece of paper to attack in the morning."
>
> —DAWN NELSON

of 32. The researchers found that those with excessive workloads and extreme time pressures had *double* the risk of GAD as those with less work and more reasonable deadlines. What's more, they also had double the risk of depression.

The researchers' conclusion? "Work stress appears to precipitate diagnosable depression and anxiety in previously healthy young workers."

In other words, you don't even have to have any particular hang-ups, repressed memories, or a rotten childhood to be turned into a hyper, always-on, never-sleeping worrywart. Your job alone can do it.

SLEEP PANIC

Panic attacks are like anxiety on steroids. They hit hard and send the mind screaming in fear, while the heart races, skips, or pounds—and sometimes all three. They can also trigger sweating, shaking, chest pain, nausea, dizziness, feeling unreal and detached from your body, and a sensation of being smothered.

Fortunately, they peak within 10 minutes.

For almost 20 percent of those who experience these attacks, the attack will occur during sleep. When it does, the individual is jerked from sleep, usually by a physical symptom such as shortness of breath.

No one knows precisely what causes those attacks, although some researchers feel that it may be related to a sensitivity to subtle increases in blood levels of carbon dioxide.

Panic attacks occur more often in women than men and typically begin in the late teens or early twenties. Fortunately, they can usually be prevented with cognitive behavior therapy or with antipanic and antidepressant medication.

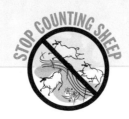

Sleep Rx for Worrywarts

When worry drives your life, studies show you're more likely to develop chronic insomnia. Here's how to prevent that—and get a good night's sleep.

REIGN IN YOUR WORK LIFE. Give your heart to your work, but be a little more stingy with your time. Decide how many hours a week is reasonable to get your work done, add 10 percent in case you're wrong, then walk away.

SWIM. Or run. Or bike. Or skate. Or skip rope with some kids on the neighborhood playground. You get the idea. Twenty minutes of aerobic exercise reroutes all the adrenaline that worry generates.

WORK ON STRESS. Since a study at the Finnish Institute of Occupational Health revealed that stressful events are twice as likely to trigger sleeping problems in those who experience anxiety, keeping a lid on daily stressors is important. Skim over the stress-reducing tips on the previous pages, pick out your favorites, and use them to do just that.

PUT WORRY ON A SCHEDULE. "In today's busy world, we don't have time to do normal worrying until the lights go out," says Mary Susan Esther, M.D., director of the Sleep Center at South Park in Charlotte, North Carolina, and president of the American Academy of Sleep Medicine. "Yet everyone needs a worry time," she adds. The trick is to schedule it on a regular basis, early in the evening—any time before 8:00 P.M.

Sit down with a stack of 3 x 5 index cards and ask yourself, "What am I worried about?" Then write down one worry on each card. When you seem to have written down your last worry, go back to the first card, reflect on the worry it describes, and give yourself a reality check.

Does the worry involve a problem that you can do something about? If not, rip up the card. If there is something you can do, write down possible actions and tuck the card into a worry box. You can give it more thought in the morning and decide what to do.

STAY OFF EBAY. In fact, shut off your computer altogether, urges Dr. Esther. A lot of people with worry insomnia are tempted to go online before bed and play computer solitaire or check eBay to see if they've won what they were bidding on. "But the computer is interactive, so you can't just watch, you have to respond," says the sleep specialist. "And that interaction is stimulating enough to keep you up half the night."

For instance, one Florida woman boots up every night around 10:00 P.M. She intends only to check her bids on eBay. Since she feels she has a sleep problem, she intends to be in bed by 11:00 P.M. But without fail, she's still online at 3:00 A.M. "What can I do?" she asks with a helpless shrug. "I just can't sleep!"

HEAD FOR THE BATHROOM. Once you've shut down the computer and had your scheduled worry session, a warm bath before bed will not only relax you, it will also adjust your body's temperature to a point that signals your brain: "Hey, honey, it's time for sleep."

HIDE THE CLOCKS. "Digital clocks blare time at you," says Dr. Esther. "It's normal to wake throughout the night, but if you look at a clock and see the time, it's likely to increase your anxiousness about not being asleep." If you need a clock to wake you in the morning, just turn its face to the wall right before bed. You'll hear it just as well.

KEEP MILK AND COOKIES WITHIN REACH. Milk contains sleep-inducing tryptophan, but you need carbs to get it into your brain. Dr. Esther likes cookies (low-fat, of course) as the carb, but you could substitute crackers if you'd prefer. There are tryptophan supplements on the market, but neither she nor the FDA recommends them; their safety is still in question.

NIX NIGHTCAPS. "Sometimes sleepless individuals will have a drink or two to help fall asleep," says Dr. Esther. "While it will shorten time falling asleep, alcohol actually causes more arousal as your body metabolizes it. The result is it shortens sleep.

"A glass of wine with dinner is okay," she adds. "But a glass afterward may have an impact on your sleep."

TREAT YOURSELF LIKE A CHILD. Create a nurturing postbath, prebed routine that's intended to help you wind down, says Dr. Esther. A little reading, a little soft music—whatever makes you feel nurtured and relaxed.

"We tend to take care of everyone else before we take care of ourselves," says Dr. Esther. "That has to change."

STOP THOSE THOUGHTS. Once you hit the sheets, worry time is over—especially about sleeping. There's a therapy trick called "thought-stopping" that works like a charm, says Dr. Esther. "If you find yourself thinking about tomorrow and saying, `It's going to be a bad day because I'm never going to sleep,' immediately think: `STOP. Don't go there. I know I've done this before. If I don't fall asleep, I'll get out of bed, flip through a magazine, but I am NOT going to focus on this stuff!'" Sounds simple, but once you try it, you'll find it works!

RESTRICT TIME IN BED TO SLEEP TIME. If you're going to bed at 10:00 P.M., sleeping from 11:30 P.M. until 2:00 A.M., tossing and turning until 4 A.M., then sleeping until 6, you've gotten 8 hours in bed but only 4½ hours of sleep. That's a huge mismatch, which can actually inhibit your sleep drive and cause insomnia all by itself. To prevent it, when you wake at 2, go read a book in the living room. Being up increases your sleep drive—which could make you sleepy enough to fall asleep when you return to bed.

SCHEDULE YOUR SLEEP TIME. "Stick with it seven days a week," says Dr. Esther. Opening your eyes at the same time every morning triggers a series of bio-chemicals that, as the day winds down, tell your body when it's time to sleep.

WORK WITH A COGNITIVE BEHAVIORAL THERAPIST. In a study at the Université Laval in Quebec, researchers measured the effects of cognitive behavioral therapy for GAD on insomnia and found that insomnia prac-tically disappeared among study participants.

What's more, in 21 other studies involving 470 patients with insomnia from a variety of causes, cognitive behavioral therapy worked just as well as sleeping pills at increasing sleep and improving sleep quality—and it was actually *better* than sleeping pills at helping study partici-pants get to sleep faster.

Despite its intimidating name, cognitive behavioral therapy—or CBT—is simply learning new information about what keeps you from sleeping (the "cognitive" part) and learning how to manipulate your behavior (the "behavioral" part) so that it doesn't. It generally takes only four or five 30-minute sessions to effect change.

Unfortunately, certified cognitive behavioral therapists are scarce. To find one, visit www.academyofct.org and click on "Find a Certified Cognitive Therapist." Fill in your Zip code on the pop-up, and a list of therapists in your area will appear. If none do, you can visit www.cbtforinsomnia.com. The Harvard researcher who demonstrated the effectiveness of CBT vs. sleeping pills has taken his study and pack-aged it into an online program. (For more information see page 30.)

SEEK A SLEEP SPECIALIST. "If you've been struggling with a sleep prob-lem for almost a month, talk to a sleep specialist," suggests Dr. Esther. "You already know what your issues are, but a sleep specialist might be helpful by prescribing an anti-anxiety medication to use for a few weeks as you get control of your worries and establish better sleep habits."

Depression

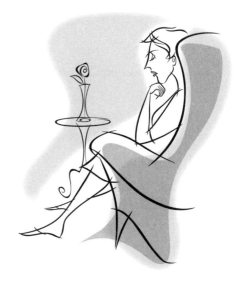

When 29-year-old actor Marty Merriweather gets up and heads toward a meeting with film producers in Los Angeles several times a week, the 30-minute trip up Route 5 and across town to their studios—which to many by this point would seem rather routine—is a major triumph of both spirit and determination.

Insomnia may be a **harbinger** of an **oncoming** episode of **depression**.

The reason? Like some 14.8 million men and women in this country, Marty lives with major depression, a nasty biochemical screwup in the brain related to serotonin and norepinephrine—two chemical neurotransmitters that affect sleep, memory, mood, energy, weight, concentration, decision making, and a host of other factors conducive to your health, happiness, and ability to function in the world.

The Cost

Unfortunately, when these neurotransmitters are thrown out of balance, the result can generate depression, which is largely identified by a gathering of symptoms that can include feelings of worthlessness, guilt, anxiety, pessimism, a sense of emptiness, a mind-numbing fatigue, a persistent sadness, and a sense of hopelessness that can easily make it difficult to see the point in getting out of bed each morning.

It's a difficult disorder. At its best, depression can rob you of the ability to feel joy. At its worst, it can rob you of your life. Up to 15 percent of those with a string of severe depressive episodes commit suicide.

In Marty's case the disease began innocently while she was in the middle of acting in three movies back to back. With millions of the studios' dollars riding on her work, the pressure was intense, the work never-ending, the deadlines firm.

Things seemed okay at first, but by the time the third film rolled around, Marty was struggling to recapture the joy that had infused her work. "I was hot," she says today. "I had worked for 10 years to get where I was and I was there—sitting where everyone else wanted to be."

She shakes her head. "I couldn't have cared less."

THE DEPRESSED BRAIN

Up to 90 percent of women with depression have one or all of the following sleep issues:

- Difficulty falling asleep
- Difficulty staying asleep
- Waking in the early morning—say, around 2 or 3 o'clock
- Less restorative sleep
- More "light" sleep
- Decreased total hours of sleep
- Disruptive dreams

Does Insomnia Cause Depression?

Most people who develop depression can frequently point to a precipitating stressor, like a divorce, job loss, medical illness, weekend binge, chronic work overload, crazy boss, financial problems, or other highly stressful situation that can knock neurotransmitters awry and trigger a chemical imbalance in the brain.

But what underlies that imbalance can be complex. Studies indicate that more than 50 percent of the risk of depression may also be due to genetic factors that can knock things out of whack, and in women—who have twice the rate of depression as men—the effects of ever

One Woman's Story

MARY SAFFORD: Sleepless in Chicago

When Mary Safford, an educational consultant based in Chicago, first became aware she was depressed, it was almost a relief. She hadn't been able to figure out why life was such a struggle—and had basically come to the conclusion that it was because she was so incompetent that she was always shooting herself in the foot.

Once the problem had been identified, however, she knew it could be solved.

At first she turned to yoga, exercise, and a diet free of alcohol, sugar, and caffeine. It made her feel better, but it wasn't enough. So she turned to therapy. She'd had a lot of early experiences that traumatized her, so in therapy she worked to understand what had happened and to integrate that new understanding into her feelings.

Again, that helped. Tremendously. But it wasn't until Mary, a Quaker, turned to her faith that she truly began to feel whole.

"The Quaker perspective is that of being in the experience and asking, changing levels of the hormones estrogen and progesterone are a wild card that leaves all the experts scratching their heads. What's particularly intriguing to researchers right now, however, is the novel idea that insomnia may actually play a role in the onset of depression.

"Insomnia is the first symptom to appear in depression and the last to go away," says Ruth Benca, M.D., Ph.D., and director of the sleep program at the University of Wisconsin-Madison. "Whether it's a first episode or a recurrence, insomnia shows up first. We don't know why. One explanation is that some of the same systems overlap in the brain, and once something disrupts those systems, you see both insomnia and depression."

`What am I to learn from this? What is being asked of me?' " says Mary. "And what I've found through my whole healing process is that if I can focus on those two questions, it keeps my focus a lot wider.

"That counteracts depression," she explains, "because what depression does is narrow your vision. You get totally focused on `What's happening to me?' And in really serious depression, people can become so focused on how bad they feel that they consider killing themselves. It's a slippery slope that can lead someone off the edge."

The support of her faith community is also important, Mary explains. "In our Quaker meeting, we have a Meeting for Healing, in which people pray together for healing that matches the will of God," she says.

"We don't necessarily say this in words. Our intention is that the person who needs healing is filled with the Holy Spirit and that her healing process follows the will of God.

"That could mean relief of symptoms, a total cure, or learning the lessons that come with illness. Or it could mean feeling strengthened and being able to thrive in the midst of a difficult situation.

"For me healing doesn't necessarily mean cure," she adds. "But it certainly means being at peace."

Amazingly, insomnia may be an early harbinger of an oncoming episode of depression. What's more, adds James P. Krainson, M.D., a sleep medicine specialist at Miami's South Florida Sleep Diagnostic Center, "treating chronic insomnia may be a way of decreasing the risk of depression."

Winter Depression

If you find yourself going to bed early, sleeping later, feeling sleepy all day, and craving waistline-bulging carbs as the days get shorter in September and October, chances are that you're trying to hibernate.

If you were a bear, it wouldn't be a problem. But since you're not, it means you likely have a mild form of depression called Winter Depression, or Seasonal Affective Disorder.

It's a problem that affects more than 11 million of us every year. Four times as many women develop it as men, and those who live in the northern United States and Canada are eight times as likely to experience it as those living farther south.

The problem is the hormone melatonin, which is produced in a specific part of your brain when the sun goes down. It's a major controlling factor in sleep, and during the low-light months of fall and winter, those of us with a tendency toward winter depression tend to produce more melatonin than others—enough to make us sleepy and sap our energy. Fortunately, exposure to bright light is the cure. It suppresses the brain's production of melatonin and helps to maintain control of our sleep cycle, energy production, and carbs.

Most of us don't get enough bright light in the winter, so researchers have developed a device called a light box that will give us what we need. The device produces an intense white light, and using it for 20 to 30 minutes every day can lift winter depression.

To find a listing of light-box manufacturers, go to the Web site for the Society for Light Treatment and Biological Rhythms at www.sltbr.org.

Beat Depression

Depression is a life-threatening disorder that seems to be triggered by stress, hormones, genetic glitches, medical conditions, medication, and maybe even the kitchen sink. Its onset is predicted by insomnia, insomnia usually accompanies it, and insomnia is usually the last symptom to disappear. Maybe that's why, as Ruth Benca, M.D., Ph.D., and director of the sleep program at the University of Wisconsin-Madison, says, "All the things that are good sleep therapy are good depression therapy, too." Here are the strategies that can help you beat both.

CHECK WITH YOUR PRIMARY-CARE PHYSICIAN. Depression can be the side effect of a laundry list of illnesses—cancer, for one; sleep apnea, for another—and medications. So if you're feeling down for any length of time, your first step is your primary-care physician.

SEE A PSYCHIATRIST. Depression can kill, and the medications frequently used to rebalance your brain chemicals can be tricky. So once your primary-care physician has ruled out medical conditions and medication as a cause of depression, even if you're comfortable with your primary physician's care, you might want to ask for a referral to a psychiatrist.

Your primary-care physician may be able to deal with depression as a temporary side effect or the everyday blues, but it's a psychiatrist who is trained in the ins and outs of major depression and its treatment, and it's a psychiatrist who is most able to suggest the treatment option that, tailored to your particular situation and combination of issues, is most likely to succeed.

THINK ABOUT THE BIG 3. The three approaches doctors usually suggest for major depression are antidepressant medication and either cognitive behavioral therapy (CBT) or interpersonal psychotherapy (IPT), says James P. Krainson, M.D., a sleep medicine specialist at Miami's South Florida Sleep Diagnostic Center.

"Most depression responds to medication," he adds. Since it's likely to be caused by a biochemical imbalance in your brain, a chemical can frequently help. Fortunately, however, depression responds well to all three treatments.

In a review of studies conducted at Vanderbilt University, researchers found that medication had a rapid and robust effect, plus it prevented the return of symptoms for as long as it was taken.

In the review, both CBT and IPT seemed to be just as effective as medication. In particular, IPT might help the individual work out personal issues, while CBT seemed to have an enduring effect that reduced the risk of future depressive episodes—a big concern among doctors.

Combined treatment with both medication and therapy seemed the best choice, the researchers concluded, since combination therapy seemed to boost the effectiveness of each.

TRY AGAIN. "Studies have shown that about half of those who start on a treatment of medication and/or therapy get some relief," says researcher George Niederehe, Ph.D., the National Institute of Mental Health's project officer for STAR *D, a nationwide series of studies that included more than 4,000 men and women diagnosed with major depressive disorder. But doctors weren't sure how to help the other half once the initial therapy had failed. Common sense told them to try another medication and see what happened, which is what many doctors did. Still, they wanted some clear direction about what helped and what didn't—or if there was another way to approach treatment altogether.

Enter the STAR *D study. Conducted in the real world among people with demanding jobs and relationships, the study has shown how to help the *other* half—the group science seemed to have left behind.

There were two key studies in STAR *D. "One study looked at how well people did if their original treatment was supplemented with a second one. The other looked at how well people did if their original medication was switched with another," says Dr. Niederehe.

In the first study, in which an original antidepressant medication that hadn't achieved complete remission of symptoms was supplemented with a second antidepressant, 1 in 3 patients achieved a remission of symptoms.

In the second study, in which patients were switched from the original antidepressant to another, 1 in 4 patients achieved a remission.

"In both cases the finding was that the move to a second treatment benefited a substantial number of patients," says Dr. Niederehe, who further explains that when thinking about treatment for depression, there are a couple of things revealed by STAR *D to keep in mind.

One is that even though the 10 medications used in STAR *D work via different mechanisms, they all worked in the same numbers of people. In other words, no one antidepressant was more effective than any other. The other is that if you begin to take a particular medication and show even a partial benefit, you should stick with that particular medication for a full 12 weeks because you may well achieve remission in that time.

On the other hand, if you show no benefit at all after eight weeks on one medication, you should talk with your doctor about switching.

The bottom line, says Dr. Niederehe, is this: "If you fail at the first treatment, don't give up. It may just be that you haven't found the right approach. Another treatment is likely to help. And by giving treatment another try, you have a good chance of complete remission."

ATTACK THE INSOMNIA. "You need to treat the insomnia at the same time as you treat the depression," says Sonia Ancoli-Israel, Ph.D., a professor of psychiatry at the University of California at San Diego. "You don't just treat the depression and then assume that the insomnia will go away on its own."

What's more, she adds, "There have been studies on depression that show that if you treat both the depression and the insomnia at the same time, concurrently, you'll get a better, faster response not only to the insomnia, but to the depression as well."

So put the basic insomnia-fighting strategies to work: Go to bed at the same time every night. Get up at the same time every morning. Walk in the noonday sun without sunglasses. Each of these strategies uses the presence or absence of light to set off a chemical reaction in your brain that ultimately affects the neurotransmitters involved in depression. It's no coincidence that light therapy alone is used to treat a specific form of depression called "winter depression" (see page 84).

If you're still not sleeping after a few days, ask your health-care provider to give you a hand, says Dr. Ancoli-Israel. "And don't let her dismiss the idea that sleep is important," she adds. "If necessary, make a separate appointment to discuss your insomnia with her."

REPORT THOUGHTS OF SUICIDE IMMEDIATELY. The idea of suicide is common in severe depression. If the thought even passes through your mind, call your doctor or 911 immediately. Severely depressed people do commit suicide.

SEE A SLEEP SPECIALIST. If you have severe depression and you can't sleep, you may want to ask your doctor for a referral to a sleep center, suggests Dr. Benca. A sleep center's specialized testing and trained scientists may be able to give you some help.

PRACTICE YOUR FAITH. A study at Duke University found that severely depressed people who put their faith at the center of their lives recovered 70 percent faster than those who did not.

SWEAT. Another Duke University study found that 30 minutes of exercise, in which you work up a sweat, is just as effective as antidepressants in reducing major depression. What's more, another study found that exercise is key to preventing relapses—a serious problem in those who have had more than one episode of depression.

HANG OUT WITH FRIENDS. In a British study, hanging out with a friend on a regular basis lifted the spirits of those with mild depression.

STRUCTURE YOUR DAY. People who have depression frequently lead unstructured lives, says Ruth Benca, M.D., P.h.D. Unfortunately, it contributes to both depression and insomnia. So put yourself on a schedule and stick to it. Eating, sleeping, working, exercising, socializing—figure out what times work for you and then carve them in stone.

IF IT SWIMS, EAT IT. Those who consume diets rich in omega-3 fatty acids, a type of fat found in cold-water fish such as salmon, are less likely to experience depression than others, reports a Dutch study. And a study in England found that pregnant women who ate 10 ounces of fish a day had half the rate of depression as women who didn't. In fact, some researchers think that the amount of depression in America is directly related to a lack of fish in our diet.

ENLIST YOUR PARTNER. A study of 84 depressed pregnant women found that those who were given two 20-minute massages a week from their partners reduced their incidence of depression by 70 percent. The researchers suspect massage boosts serotonin levels and reduces levels of stress hormones.

STAY OUT ALL NIGHT. But only once, and only with your doctor's approval and support. This is a bit tricky, since it can make depression worse. But the odd thing is that depriving yourself of sleep for one night—and no more than that—has been shown to lift depression for as long as a month. Researchers don't know how it works, but they suspect that one night of sleep deprivation may reset your sleep clock.

TAKE CARE OF BUSINESS. In London, researchers at King's College have spent three decades looking into the effect of workloads, deadlines, and other job-related stressors on nearly a thousand young working adults. They've found that these types of jobs demand nearly double the risk of depression in women.

If you find yourself getting depressed at the thought of going in to work because of the workload or time demands, talk to your employer and try to negotiate a saner workload, more realistic deadlines, or assistance from other colleagues. If your boss isn't interested, put the word out to friends: You're looking for a new job.

A WOMAN'S BEST FRIEND, TOO. When people without pets played with a dog for just a few minutes a day as part of a University of Missouri study, levels of the brain chemicals serotonin and oxytocin—both mood elevators—rose. You don't have to own a dog to get these benefits, either. Volunteer at an animal shelter to walk a dog, or just pet your neighbor's whenever it trots by.

EAT A BOWL OF FORTIFIED CEREAL EVERY DAY. Or take a multivitamin. Either will provide you with 400 micrograms of folate, a B vitamin that is known to lift depression. Folate and other vitamins help maintain nerve and blood cells, which are used in brain reactions and are essential for the production and function of a number of mood-boosting brain chemicals. And a study published in the *Annals of Clinical Psychiatry* found that folate actually helps enhance the effectiveness of antidepressants.

STAY ON MEDS. Depressive episodes tend to recur. To reduce the risk of relapse, doctors recommend that you stay on medication for six months to a year even though you may be feeling normal again.

STAY ALERT. Insomnia can herald the return of depression before you're even aware of it. If you start having sleep problems again, schedule an appointment with your doctor. Early detection and treatment can minimize its effect on your life—and even head it off.

Work Schedules

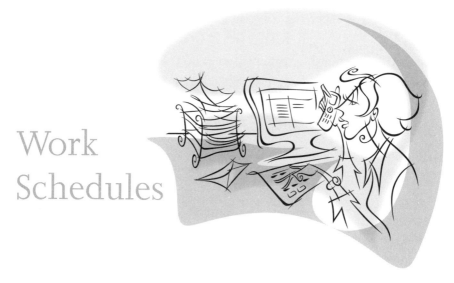

Doctors, nurses, firefighters, truck drivers, police officers, security personnel, EMTs, airline crews—we are clearly in debt to all of those many men and women who are willing to work around the clock to keep us healthy, safe, and in motion.

But recent research indicates that these shift workers—and society as a whole—may be paying a much higher price for their 24-hour service than anyone could have guessed.

Here's why.

9 to 5 is hard enough. But what about the **25 million** of us who **work around** the **clock?**

Too Many Consequences

Studies show that 85 percent of police officers, 80 percent of regional pilots, and 48 percent of air-traffic controllers nod off on the job. And a frightening 41 percent of medical workers admit they've made fatigue-related errors. In one survey alone, 19 percent report "worsening" a patient's condition. What's more, the Exxon Valdez grounding, the space shuttle *Challenger* accident, and the Three

One Woman's Story

JASMINKA STEGIC: Sleepless in Los Angeles

Walking out of Cedars Sinai Medical Center into the morning sunshine on a busy Los Angeles street, Jasminka Stegic, a critical-care nurse practitioner, is exhausted.

"My shift ends at 7:00 A.M., and by 7:30 I can hardly keep my eyes open," she admits. "I love what I do. But I *don't* love the night shift."

Fortunately, Jasminka lives only a 10-minute walk from the hospital, so she doesn't have to drive, a problem for many shift workers. A month-long study of 895 nurses at Grand Valley State University in Michigan recently found that almost two-thirds of the nurses struggled to stay awake at work, while nearly 80 percent of the nurses reported at least one incident of drowsy driving during the month after getting off work.

That's a problem to which Jasminka can relate. When she worked the night shift at a hospital in Texas, she lived 20 miles away. And she can still remember the sound of those rumble strips at the road's edge that warned her when, exhausted after a long night, she was driving off the road.

Now, however, her walk lets her take a deep breath and re-orient herself to the world. "I go home, take a shower, and eat a high-carb meal—usually

Mile Island nuclear accident have all been blamed, at least in part, on fatigue related to sleep loss.

Besides the negative consequences resulting on the job, shift workers are feeling the effects of their schedules. A study of 437 day workers and 246 rotating shift workers at the Universidad de Buenos Aires in Argentina found that shift workers have seriously lower levels of serotonin, a hormone that plays a role in regulating sleep and mood, than their day-working counterparts. Unfortunately, lower levels of serotonin are associated with anger, depression, and anxiety, as well as poor sleep.

toast with butter and jelly or cereal and a banana," says Jasminka. She knows that carbs will make her even sleepier, and she's found that she's more likely to stay asleep longer when her body's got some to process.

But daytime sleep is still tough because Jasminka lives in an apartment building. Elevators are always opening and closing, discharging groups of people who don't realize that someone nearby may be trying to sleep. So before she gets into bed, Jasminka places earplugs in her ears. Then she pulls special light-blocking drapes across her windows and hops into bed.

"I only stay asleep for two to five hours after working a night shift," she says. "And that sleep is fragmented. So when I wake up, my head hurts and I feel beat up. I lie around hoping I'll fall back asleep."

That generally doesn't seem to happen, so eventually she'll get up and read or take her dog for a walk.

"I don't do much before my shift starts again," she admits.

Once it's time for work, however, Jasminka starts to rev up for the night ahead. She drinks a large double espresso from Starbucks on her way to work, then drinks lattes on the job. At the hospital the nature of critical-care work keeps her pumped with adrenaline, and during a shift break she avoids the heavy carbs that would make her sleepy.

"I love my job," she repeats firmly. But even she admits she'll love it even more when a slot on the day shift opens up.

Another study, conducted by Harvard Medical School—this one of more than 78,000 women who worked rotating night shifts over a 10-year period—found that shift work significantly increased a woman's risk of breast cancer.

A second team of Harvard researchers studied the same group, and they found that women who worked a rotating night shift at least three nights per month for 15 or more years had an increased risk of colorectal cancer.

> "I count my breaths up to four, then start over at one, concentrating on the breaths and nothing else. That way, no scary thoughts, no old worries or concerns about what I have to do the next day can squeeze their way into my mind and keep me awake."
>
> —DELIE REX

And a third team of Harvard researchers studied more than 53,000 women who worked rotating shifts and found that night work increased the women's risk of endometrial cancer by 47 percent—and actually doubled the risk of endometrial cancer in obese shift workers.

It's this type of research that led the World Health Organization late in 2007 to classify shift work as a "probable" cause of cancer—a position that the American Cancer Society indicates it is likely to follow.

WHEN TO LOOK FOR A DAY JOB

- You feel tired all the time.
- You're grumpy.
- You make frequent mistakes.
- You worry you'll nod off behind the wheel.
- You're missing watching your kids grow up.

The Tyranny of Hard Wiring

Most of the 25 million hardworking American women who work rotating night shifts get between five to seven hours less sleep each week than their nonshift friends and neighbors, says sleep researcher Kar-Ming Lo, M.D., FCCP, a critical-care specialist in the Akron, Ohio, Summa Health System.

It's a seemingly insignificant deficit, but two hours of sleep loss, studies report, have the same effect on your brain as knocking back two or three 12-ounce beers. It's also an amount that week after week, year after year, may build up to a huge effect.

Most workers try to catch up on weekends, but how much that helps is a matter of intense debate and millions of research dollars. Given the complexity of individual biology and the variables of each individual work situation, soon-to-be-released studies from the University of Pennsylvania suggest that recovery from sleep deprivation may not be as simple as sleeping an extra four hours on Saturday and Sunday to make up for the four you lost during the week.

So why aren't our shift workers getting the sleep they need?

"There are three main reasons," says Dr. Lo.

For one thing, our bodies are hardwired to be alert and active during the day and sleepy at night. But when you sleep during the day, many of the brain chemicals that keep the brain asleep in response to darkness are simply not released—or not released in the amounts you need for good sleep and optimal health.

As a result, says Dr. Lo, shift workers miss out on a portion of the restorative sleep you need to build and repair the body. Shift workers also get less of the other types of sleep, which affect mood, memory, and the ability to make quick decisions.

A second reason shift workers aren't getting proper sleep is that sleeping during the day runs against the grain of society. You can come home and lie down to sleep at 9 or 10 o'clock every morning, but the rest of the world goes on. Dogs bark, trash haulers pick up the recycling, hedge trimmers keep the world neat.

What's more, since most people don't understand the biological importance of sleep, your *need* to sleep may not be respected—even within your own family. Your children may wake you and demand attention as they run in the door after school at 3 o'clock, or your husband may try to initiate sex on the one day all week you have to sleep in. Studies reveal that shift work actually increases the risk of divorce by 57 percent.

It's a tough way to make a living.

What's really diabolical, however, is the fact that over the course of a week, the shift workers' biological clocks will begin to adjust. That sounds like a good thing, but come the weekend, many shift workers try to be more a part of the family and live life on the family's schedule. One mother may get only a few hours of sleep, then get up and go to her daughter's T-ball game. She'll come home and nap, get up again, make dinner, and eat with her family. Another mom may cut short her sleep to take a child to the doctor's, then spend a little time shopping at the mall. She'll nap during the afternoon, then make dinner and eat with the family.

Soon-to-be-released studies from the University of Pennsylvania suggest that recovery from sleep deprivation may not be as simple as sleeping an extra four hours on Saturday and Sunday to make up for the four you lost during the week.

Unfortunately, says Dr. Lo, those innocent attempts to participate in family life on the family's schedule is enough to throw all the adjustments her biological clock made the week before into disarray. The result is that she'll feel cranky, exhausted, and sleep deprived for the first two days of the next week—the time it will take her body to readjust.

You think jet lag is bad?

"The lag from shift work is worse," says Dr. Lo.

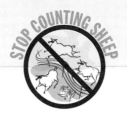

How to Get Restorative Sleep

Shift work twirls the dials on your body's biological clock until it can't tell when it should wake you up and when it should let you sleep. And although there's no single magic plan that's right for everyone, there is agreement among sleep researchers that the following strategies will help you get a good night's sleep. Here's how to get started.

GET YOUR PARTNER ON BOARD. Shift work is tough on the entire family. Make sure your partner knows how it will affect him—increased parental responsibilities and household tasks, less time with you—*before* you sign on for night or rotating work.

GIVE YOUR BODY A THREE-DAY WARNING. If you're headed toward a major change in work schedule, begin to alter your sleep time three days in advance.

Let's say your usual shift is 5:00 P.M. to 1:00 A.M. and you're moving to an 11:00 P.M. to 7:00 A.M. schedule. If you usually sleep from 3:00 to 11:00 A.M., postpone your bedtime to 5:00 A.M. and sleep until 1:00 P.M. on the first day of the transition.

On day 2 postpone your bedtime to 7:00 A.M. and sleep until 3:00 P.M. On day 3 postpone bedtime to 8:00 A.M. and sleep until 4:00 P.M. On day 4 you'll begin the new 11:00 P.M. to 7:00 A.M. shift. That day sleep from 9:00 A.M. until 5:00 P.M.—and on every day thereafter.

MAINTAIN A SCHEDULE. Keep the same sleep/wake schedule on your at-home days as on your workdays, says sleep specialist Kar-Ming Lo, M.D. It will help your body understand when you need to be alert and when you need to sleep.

WORK CLOCKWISE. If you work rotating shifts, ask your manager to schedule succeeding shifts so that a new shift starts later than the last one, recommends the American Academy of Sleep Medicine. If you've just finished a 3:00 to 11:00 P.M. shift, for example, you'll be more alert and sleep better if the next shift you work is 11:00 P.M. to 7:00 A.M.

GET OUTDOORS. Once you wake up, get outside. Take a walk and sit in the sun. The sun will cue your biological clock that it's time to be alert.

PASS UP OPPORTUNITIES. Shift work stresses the body big-time. It puts your health at risk and denies you time with your family. Even if you need extra money, think twice about accepting an opportunity to work overtime or extra hours or skip vacations. The price may be higher than the added income.

GET A PICKUP. Two-thirds of shift workers report driving drowsy after a shift—and drowsy driving is the direct cause of an estimated 1,550 deaths every year. Take the bus, hire a cab, have someone better rested than you are pick you up after your shift and take you home.

MAKE SLEEP A FAMILY EFFORT. Discuss your sleep needs with kids, says Dr. Lo. Tell the kids that "Mom's working hard and she works nights." Then ask that they not go into your room unless it's an emergency. And be sure to specify precisely what is—and what is not—an emergency.

STICK TO PERRIER. If you feel like a nightcap—morningcap?—make it water. Although alcohol may seem to relax you so you can get to sleep more quickly, what it actually does is disrupt your sleep later in the night. As a result, you get less sleep and sleep that's less than refreshing.

FORGET THE QUICK FIX. There isn't any, although there are plenty of people around who will sell you one. One example: Sales of the herb valerian, which has historically been used to aid sleep, have reached more than a million dollars a year. Yet a review of 37 sleep studies reveals that it doesn't do a thing.

USE ROOM-DARKENING DRAPES. They are lined with a heavy light-blocking fabric that will give you your best shot at convincing your brain it's dark and therefore time to sleep. Use them in the bedroom and wherever else you might wander during a rest period.

FORGET THE EARLY-BIRD SPECIAL. Don't stop at the store for early-bird specials or watch late-late-late-night shows or early morning news shows once you get home, says Dr. Lo. Hit the hay.

NAP. A 20- to 30-minute nap just before reporting for the night shift can increase your alertness on the job.

CREATE A COCOON OF QUIET. Close the windows, turn off the phone, wear earplugs, and use white noise, says Dr. Lo. Running a bedroom air-conditioning unit during the summer or a fan in winter will mute outside distractions like trash haulers and slamming doors.

LIVE CLOSE TO YOUR JOB. A long commute steals sleep, says Dr. Lo. A short one facilitates it.

GET FIXED. If you have the option of working a fixed shift—that is, the same shift each and every evening or night—go for it. You'll feel and sleep better.

GET HELP. If you feel as though you're walking under water all the time, ask your doctor if a prescription medication, melatonin, or bright-light therapy might help.

INFLUENCE WORK POLICIES. If your employer knew that a 26-minute nap could double your productivity, don't you think he'd make naps an approved corporate policy and figure out how to make nap time available? He probably would—especially if you've been complaining that you're tired. So do some research—you can start at www.sleepeducation.com—and develop some suggestions that will help you feel less fatigued and solve a problem or two for your employer. Who knows? You may end up getting a promotion along with a nap!

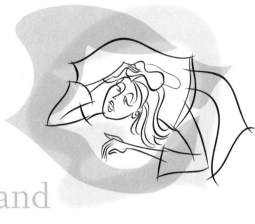

Hormones and Biological Changes

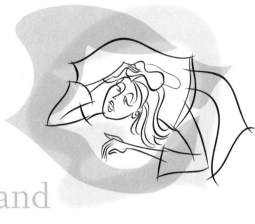

> **67 percent of women lose sleep** during their menstrual cycle every **month.**

Hormones.

Male neurologists, gynecologists, and sleep medicine specialists may think of them simply as messenger molecules that zip instructions from one part of the body to another.

Female neurologists, gynecologists, and sleep medicine specialists, however, know them for who they really are: the messengers from hell. Whether those little molecular mavericks are making us toss and turn with premenstrual insomnia or keeping us bolt upright at 3:00 A.M. during the hormonal roller coaster of perimenopause, these messengers can disrupt the most well-balanced woman and send her tumbling into a sleepless void from which she returns exhausted, stressed, and desperately searching for Starbucks.

Fortunately, even the messengers from hell can be whipped into shape. Here's how.

Menstrual Insomnia: Hijacking Your Body's Ability to Heal

Every sexually active woman not on birth control pills knows that three things are going to happen each and every month:

1. She'll eat more chocolate than either she or God intended.
2. She'll wonder if it's possible she's pregnant.
3. She's going to lose some sleep.

The problem, of course, is hormones. According to a poll by the National Sleep Foundation, 67 percent of women who menstruate toss and turn for two or three days during every menstrual cycle—a number that Kathryn Lee, Ph.D., a sleep researcher at the University of California, San Francisco, who conducted the poll, finds entirely believable.

Although many women will have trouble sleeping due to bloating, breast tenderness, backaches, or pelvic aches and pains during their periods, says Dr. Lee, "those women who have regular cycles and who monitor their sleep frequently find that they also have insomnia a day or two before menstruation begins.

"It kind of gets lost in the tossing and turning at the beginning of menstruation unless you keep a sleep log," she adds. "Then it jumps right out."

Premenstrual insomnia, as doctors call it, seems to be associated with a rapid drop in the hormone progesterone. "Progesterone is a soporific, a sedative-type drug that your body gives you every month when you ovulate," says Dr. Lee. "Then, just before your period, its production either slows to a trickle or falls dramatically."

> *"I keep crossword puzzles from the newspaper under my bed. When I wake up at 3:00 A.M., I turn on the light, pick one up, and work on it. I'm off to sleep within a relatively short time."*
>
> —DIANE MICHAUD

If the drop is gradual, she claims, your sleep will probably be a little troubled. When progesterone plummets, however, you're likely to find yourself up at 3:00 A.M. asking the dog if he wants to go for a walk.

Monthly Jet Lag

Premenstrual insomnia not only affects your ability to sleep, it also seems to affect the *quality* of your sleep.

"Normally, we start REM sleep"—the sleep in which your brain is most active—"about 90 minutes after we fall asleep," explains Dr. Lee. "But when women ovulate and progesterone makes their temperature go up, REM sleep occurs earlier in the sleep cycle, within 60 minutes." As a result, you skip over or significantly reduce the deep-sleep stage that usually occurs right before REM sleep.

"It's very similar to what happens in people who are depressed or jet-lagged," explains Dr. Lee.

THE CRAZIES

Every month a small group of women go down for the count in the week preceding their periods.

They have difficulty sleeping and experience a range of negative moods that can include anxiety, panic attacks, crying jags, anger, irritability, and a sense of being totally crazy and out of control. A few days after their periods start, the women bounce back.

Although these symptoms are reminiscent of PMS, they are generally more severe. The sadness, hopelessness, and mood swings can disrupt relationships and bring some women to the brink of suicide.

The disorder is called premenstrual dysphoric disorder (PMDD), and it is one nasty problem. No one knows the exact cause, but a team of researchers at the University of North Carolina at Chapel

Unfortunately, that deep-sleep stage is where your body's repair mechanisms swing into play. Cells increase their production of proteins that repair damage from stress and ultraviolet radiation. The immune system powers up. Metabolic functions determine ratios of fat and muscle. "And that first deep sleep of the night is where you secrete this big bolus of growth hormone," says Dr. Lee. "In children it triggers growth. In adults it heals."

Intrigued with what her studies uncovered, Dr. Lee wondered how premenstrual insomnia was affecting women with PMS, who, along with insomnia, also experience anxiety, depression, irritability, food cravings, and all the other aggravations that define the condition. Would they experience less deep sleep than other women? Would deep sleep occur at a later time?

The answer was startling. When Dr. Lee finished the study and checked her data, she found that women with PMS had no deep sleep at all. None.

Hill recently found that women who develop this disorder frequently have a genetic glitch that may make them particularly sensitive to reproductive hormones like estrogen. Conversely, the researchers also found that women who do *not* develop the disorder may have a genetic variant that protects them from it.

These discoveries may well lead to an effective treatment for PMDD. In the meantime, the good news is that PMDD predictably occurs for a limited time, and it is mitigated by daily exercise, adequate rest, and a diet free of salt, sugar, alcohol, and caffeine. A diet rich in whole grains, vegetables, and fruit is helpful, and antidepressants called selective serotonin-reuptake inhibitors (SSRIs) can reduce symptoms when taken 14 days prior to the onset of a period.

"It wasn't just when they were premenstrual," says Dr. Lee regretfully. "I wanted to find that they had had some good, normal sleep at least sometime. But I didn't. Their sleep looked like that of the jet-lagged and the depressed—all month long."

Your Sleep/Menstrual Log

In women who have regular periods, insomnia tends to occur on a regular basis as well. Try keeping track of your sleep and menstrual symptoms for two or three cycles, suggests Dr. Lee. Then look at your log and see if you find yourself tossing and turning at the same time every month. If you do, it's easy enough to prevent. Check out the tips that begin on page 106.

Here are the questions you should be asking yourself. Make photocopies of this page or record your answers in a journal on a daily basis for three months.

❑ **Time you went to bed:** _____

❑ **How long to fall asleep:** _____

❑ **Hours slept:** _____

❑ **Time you woke up:** _____

❑ **How you felt when you woke up:** _____

_____

_____

❑ **Any symptoms:** _____

_____

_____

❑ **Any stress:** _____

❑ **Period: yes/no** _____

PMS R.I.P.

Not every woman who has premenstrual insomnia has premenstrual syndrome (PMS), but most women with PMS certainly seem to have insomnia.

Symptoms usually start five days before menstruation and end within four days afterward. They can include:

- Depression
- Anxiety
- Crying spells
- Poor concentration

- Food cravings
- Tender breasts
- Bloating
- Pain

PMS can be a disruptive condition and in some cases requires medication from your doctor. But in many cases it also yields to relatively simple remedies. Here are a few.

EXERCISE. Thirty minutes of brisk walking, swimming, or cycling every day can block pain, reduce fatigue, and lift depression.

SUPPLEMENTS. Talk with your doctor about supplementing your diet with a vitamin B complex, vitamin E, and calcium. All seem to play a part in reducing PMS symptoms.

ANTIDEPRESSANTS. Taken two weeks before symptoms start or throughout the menstrual cycle, these drugs may be helpful with symptoms related to mood.

IBUPROFEN. Although NSAIDs (non-steroidal anti-inflammatory drugs) like ibuprofen can sometimes cause stomach problems, they are top-notch pain reducers. They should not be used with diuretics. Together the two can cause kidney problems.

ORAL CONTRACEPTIVES. Some of the newer types that prevent periods may help prevent PMS as well. Ask for your doctor's opinion.

Beat Monthly Insomnia

No woman should have to toss and turn every month according to the whims of Mother Nature. Here's how to work with your body to get a good night's sleep.

PRIORITIZE IT. "Sleep should be considered as much of an important factor as things like diet, stress, exercise, and smoking," says Margaret Moline, Ph.D., former head of the sleep center at Weill Cornell Medical College in New York. Unfortunately, most of us don't realize how pivotal it is to our health, particularly during our monthly cycles. "A lot of women don't remember the last time they didn't have a sleep debt," says Dr. Moline. "I see them falling asleep every morning on the 7:00 A.M. Metro North into New York."

Being alert at that time of the morning is part of your body's natural rhythm, she explains. If you're falling asleep instead, it means you're not getting the sleep your body needs.

LOG IT. "The first step against insomnia is to develop a sleep log," says Dr. Moline. That way, you can tell whether there's a link between menstrual-cycle symptoms and sleep, between relationships and sleep, between work and sleep, between hormone fluctuations and sleep—in fact, between anything and sleep. (See "Your Sleep/Menstrual Log" on page 104.)

STOP IT. If your sleep log reveals that you have insomnia every month at the same time, ask your doctor to prescribe a sleeping pill, says Dr. Lee. Then take the medication proactively on the two or three nights when you know you won't sleep.

TAKE ADVANTAGE. On the other hand, if you're already taking another medication that has drowsiness as a side effect, ask your doctor if you can take that drug an hour before bed instead of whenever you've been taking it. A side effect like drowsiness can work against you during the day but *for* you at night.

MAKE A SLEEP SCHEDULE. Sticking to a sleep schedule that has you getting up in the morning and going to bed at the same time every day—yes, even while your period makes you feel like spending the day in bed—will also increase your ability to fall asleep.

CONSIDER ORAL CONTRACEPTIVES. Studies suggest that women who use oral contraceptives have less cycle-related insomnia. You should discuss the possibility of switching to oral contraceptives with your doctor if you regularly suffer from this monthly sleeplessness.

PAY ATTENTION TO BASICS. Increase the likelihood you'll sleep by creating a soothing environment. Make your sleep area a comfortable, dark place in which you feel safe. Keep soothing teas and herbal hot packs within reach.

WATCH OUT FOR WILD CARDS. "Some women may have other conditions that worsen during their cycle," says Dr. Moline, and any associated sleepiness may become exaggerated.

"There's some thinking that it might be related to the changes in blood volume during your cycle," she explains. When blood volume increases, your blood levels of medication may drop outside the therapeutic window. Again, keeping a log of your symptoms—including those related to your condition—will help identify the problem. And once you share the information with your doctor, you're only a step away from a solution.

NIBBLE. Menstruating women sometimes get so hungry they seem to eat every couple of hours. If you're hungry close to bedtime, however, just take a bite or two of something light, like a cracker.

CHANNEL YOUR THOUGHTS. Focus on things you love, like the flowers you might put in the garden next spring or taking your kids to see the ocean for the first time. This is not the time to work out problems.

DON'T PUT UP WITH TWITCHY LEGS. See your doctor if you are bothered by tingly or creepy-crawly legs. Women with heavy periods seem to be predisposed to restless legs syndrome (RLS), but this irritating condition can be treated. A blood test will help your doctor determine how much extra iron and folate your body requires during your period to keep your legs calm. (For more information see "Restless Legs" on page 184.)

KILL THE PAIN. If pelvic pain keeps you up during your period, talk to your doctor about taking an over-the-counter NSAID (non-steroidal anti-inflammatory drug) like ibuprofen, plus a vitamin B complex and magnesium supplement. And don't forget the old remedies of a heating pad or sex to relieve the pain. You can also often block the chemicals that produce pain with a daily aerobic workout.

FRISK YOUR OTCS. We know to avoid coffee and tea six hours before bed because the caffeine will keep us up. But many of us don't stop to think about what's in the over-the-counter drugs we use. Since caffeine also boosts the analgesic effects of aspirin, for example, it's frequently dropped into popular over-the-counter remedies advertised for pain relief during menstruation. That's fine—just as long as you use it during the morning and early afternoon. Otherwise, it can interfere with your sleep as effectively as a cup of coffee.

You might want to avoid over-the-counter drugs with antihistamines added in as well, says Dr. Lee. Especially those that have Benadryl. "They may work for men who weigh 50 pounds more than you do," she explains, "but because of the difference in body weight, many women who take them feel hung over the next morning."

Perimenopause: The 24/7 Woman

When Frisca Yan-Go wakes up beside her husband at 3:00 A.M. in their Los Angeles bedroom, her efficient mind is likely to begin popping with creative approaches that will meet the challenges she left sitting on her desk back at the UCLA Medical Center. But unlike the rest of us, she won't waste her energy by tossing, turning, and worrying about whether or not she'll remember all those brilliant thoughts the next morning. Instead, she'll calmly reach over to her nightstand, pick up a voice recorder, dictate a few words, then slide gently back into sleep.

As a neurologist and psychiatrist, as well as the medical director of the UCLA Sleep Disorders Center, Frisca L. Yan-Go, M.D., has a distinct

20 FOODS THAT MAKE YOU SLEEPY

Foods that rank high on the Glycemic Index will help you fall asleep in *half* the time you normally do if eaten four hours before bed. Since foods ranked high on the index—which is basically a scale of 1 to 100—cause a steep rise in blood sugar, they are not recommended for those with diabetes. Here are the snoozers:

Food	Value	Food	Value
Golden Grahams	71	Vanilla wafers	77
Bagel, plain	72	Grape-Nuts Flakes	80
Corn chips	72	Jelly beans	80
Watermelon	72	Pretzels	81
Honey	73	Rice cakes	82
Mashed potatoes	73	Cornflakes	84
Saltine crackers	74	Rice, instant	91
Graham crackers	74	Red baked potato	93
French fries	76	French bread	95
Frozen waffles	76	Tofu frozen dessert	115

advantage over the rest of us. For one thing, she knows what's going on in her mind and why it woke her up. For another, she has a whole bag of little tricks to shut it down and send it back to sleep.

Those tricks are particularly important during perimenopause. Some 59 percent of women between the ages of 35 and 55 won't get much sleep in the 4- to 8-year period prior to menopause that's generally referred to as perimenopause. In fact, researchers say that this group of women is more likely to experience insomnia than any other.

Unfortunately, the closer women get to menopause itself, the less they sleep. According to a 2007 National Sleep Foundation poll, by the

"When I'm a little freaked out and I can't settle down, I ask my husband to read to me when we go to bed. I rarely make it past the third page."
—JILL POTTER

WHAT IS PERIMENOPAUSE?

Perimenopause frequently stretches over a period of 10 years and includes five sometimes overlapping phases, says endocrinologist Jerilynn C. Prior, M.D., scientific director of the Centre for Menstrual Cycle and Ovulation Research at the University of British Columbia. And nobody seems to get much sleep through any of them.

The first two phases begin somewhere in the 40s, when women are still menstruating regularly. Phase 1 includes increased cramping, heavier flow, more intense premenstrual symptoms, and more frequent insomnia. Night sweats will begin in about one-third of women in this age group, says Dr. Prior, while severe migraine headaches and nausea are common. Phase 2 is more intense and may include hot flushes during the day as well as night sweats.

time women actually stop menstruating, somewhere between the ages of 45 and 51, a full 61 percent will report that they can't get to sleep or stay asleep several nights each and every week.

What's Going On

A lot of tossing and turning. Surveys indicate that roughly 57 percent of us can't sleep because of hot flushes, anxiety, depression, and chronic insomnia, while another 43 percent have a sleep disorder such as obstructed breathing, narcolepsy, or restless legs syndrome (see Sleep Disorders chapter beginning on page 180). Hot flushes alone cause women approaching menopause to briefly rouse 100 times a night—around three times more than a woman who is not.

Yet as seemingly unrelated as these challenges are, new research shows that they appear to share one thing in common: They are all

---

Phase 3 generally begins around age 47 and is marked by the beginning of an irregular flow. Night sweats may be better or worse, while daytime hot flushes become common for the 80 percent of women who will get them. A heavy flow and fatigue characterize this phase, which will generally last about four years.

Phase 4 is when things really get wild. Its beginning is signaled by your first skipped period, and from then on, you can't count on much of anything. Flow can be light or heavy, present or not, and appear or disappear on a whim. Cramps, night sweats, and hot flushes may intensify.

Phase 5 is one solid year without a period. Night sweats and daytime flushing intensify. Sleep is a gift.

Fortunately, postmenopausal life is just around the corner. And life after hormonal swings is good. Very, very good.

initiated or otherwise affected by imbalances in various hormones that are regulated by the body's biological clock in the brain's hypothalamus—the SNC.

"The SNC is where you have the axis for the sleep/wake cycle *and* the axis for all the endocrine glands that affect monthly reproductive rhythms," says Dr. Yan-Go. "They're all linked together like an orchestra," so when one cycle is out of whack, it tends to sideswipe the others as well. When perimenopause arrives

THE SLEEP DIET

Sleep yourself thin?

No, not quite. But an amazing study of 68,000 women conducted at Harvard Medical School reveals that women who sleep five hours a night are 32 percent more likely to gain 30 pounds or more as they get older than women who sleep seven hours or more.

Common sense says that someone who's awake and running around should be using up more calories than someone who's in bed. Running around should make them skinnier, right? But the study, conducted over a 16-year period, reveals that even when the women who slept longer ate more, they still gained less than women who slept less.

It's true that the group that slept longer also tended to exercise a little more. And it could be, admitted the researchers, that people who are a bit sleep deprived could metabolize calories less efficiently than those who are better rested.

But no one knows for sure. Until they do, think twice before you cut back on sleep.

Over the long haul, it may make you fat.

with its roller-coaster ride of hormonal ups and downs, the entire orchestra gets out of sync, says Dr. Yan-Go, and disrupted sleep is frequently the result (see "What *Is* Perimenopause?" on page 110).

"The best sleep we ever get is between age nine and menarchy," she adds ruefully. "After that, it's all ups and downs."

The 3:00 A.M. Wake-Up Call

Although more than half of us aren't sleeping, studies have shown that most perimenopausal women can *get* to sleep, they just can't *stay* that way. Instead, they wake intermittently throughout the night or in the wee hours of the morning.

And sometimes women aren't even aware of how often they wake, says neurologist Hrayr P. Attarian, M.D., director of the University of Vermont sleep center. "But if you're falling asleep during the day when you don't want to, or if you wake up after a good night's sleep and feel as though you haven't slept at all, then you should be talking to your physician."

One Woman's Story

Slipping out the side door onto the old Victorian porch that circles her house, a barefoot Johanna Rogers pulls a shawl over her nightgown and answers the quiet "Meow!" of her cat.

"Hey, sweet girl," she croons softly.

The night is cool, and as usual, Jo can't sleep. So she's come outside to share the summer night with the cat, sip a cognac, and light one of the two—okay, three—cigarettes she allows herself each day.

"I've had sleep issues all my life," says Jo when asked why she's up. "I dream a lot, and sometimes my dreams have been so vivid they're like an alternative existence. Sometimes I'm not even sure if I'm awake or not. It's disturbing."

Jo accepted the occasional insomnia her dreams brought until, at age 35, she was pregnant with her second child. "I was working full-time and had gotten a cold," Jo explains. "I couldn't take cold medicines, because I was pregnant, so I had to sleep sitting up for the last trimester so I could breathe. On top of that, we were living in a house just uphill from a railroad, and freight trains would roar by the house 40 times a night."

She grimaces in memory. Once her baby was born, however, things didn't get much better. "My first child had been easy," Jo explains. "But my second was cranky until 11:00 P.M. I'd feed him; he'd sleep for two hours; then I'd feed him again at 2. My husband would get up and feed him at 5." A couple of hours later the baby would be up and fussing. A year later he had settled down, and a year after that, Jo and her husband sold the house by the tracks—moving to the old Victorian.

By then, however, Jo had moved up in the corporate world and a new guy with a briefcase full of ambition was trying to knock her out of her job. He wanted to replace her with one of his cronies, and his power games became a daily issue. Eventually, a review of the day's moves and countermoves, accompanied by cognac and a cigarette, became a nightly occurrence. Sleep was iffy.

Then, when her oldest son was in fourth grade and her youngest in kindergarten, Jo's mother developed colon cancer.

The older woman's doctor said her mom had only a few months to live, and Jo and her sister were determined to make it possible for their mother to die at home. Jo's sister, who lived nearby, took a leave of absence from her job and nursed the older woman five days a week. Jo, who was her family's breadwinner and lived five hours away by car, relieved her on weekends.

It was a grueling way to live. Jo dodged power plays weekdays in her office, tried to do her job, then went home, helped the kids with homework and her husband with dinner, worked her youngest through 90 minutes of bedtime rituals, and called her sister to lend moral support.

Friday night she would drive five hours through rush-hour traffic to her mom's, then feed her, bathe her, soothe her increasing confusion, and clean her up a thousand times until her sister came back Sunday evening. At 6:00 P.M. Sunday, Jo hit the highways for the five-hour drive home—and the Monday morning power games at the office.

"By then I was in therapy once a week," says Jo. "Eighteen months later my mom died, perimenopause hit, I got depressed, and sleep was impossible." Jo's therapist told her she needed an antidepressant, which helped. As did quitting her job. And exercise at a nearby pool practically saved her life.

But nothing alleviated the insomnia—at least, not completely. Eventually, Jo accepted the fact that her sleep pattern was different from that of her friends, and that despite depression and perimenopause, she would get the sleep she needed.

"I used to wake up and be upset about it," she says. "But now I wake up, read for an hour, go back to sleep, get up at 6:15 to see my youngest off to school, then go back to sleep for another 45 minutes.

"I may not sleep the way everyone else does," she adds, "but I've relaxed into the fact that this is what works for me."

The type of insomnia that causes you to wake through the night or in the early morning hours can be caused by both external and internal factors, explains Dr. Yan-Go. Externally, you may have to go to the bathroom or you may simply be too hot or too cold. Or you may experience a hot flash or perhaps its chilly aftermath. Throw the covers off, doze, realize you're freezing, and pull the covers back up. If you're perimenopausal, you know the routine.

"When things get really tough at work, I can't sleep. I just lie there in the dark and keep going over and over and over all my projects. I've learned, however, that if I get up and make a hot cup of chamomile tea—from the flower buds, not that stuff they sell in bags—I'll be sound asleep within the hour."

—SUSAN MILLER

But insomnia caused by internal factors is less straightforward. Generally, says Dr. Yan-Go, when you wake in the middle of the night, it's because something has bubbled up from your subconscious.

The mind is very active during REM sleep, she explains, but when it actually wakes you up, it's usually involved in processing one or the other of two kinds of events: the ones that happened most recently and the ones from your past that are the most intense.

"Generally, you wake up and you just don't know why," says Dr. Yan-Go. "It may be that 5 o'clock meeting you had with your boss, or like my husband, it may be the memory of something that happened during wartime."

For recent events Dr. Yan-Go is pragmatic. If she wakes up and recalls an unfinished report left on her

"The best sleep we ever get is between age 9 and menarchy," says a rueful Frisca L. Yan-Go, M.D., medical director of the UCLA Sleep Disorders Center. "After that, it's all ups and downs."

desk at work, rather than worrying about it and letting it disrupt her sleep, she'll pick up the voice recorder on her night table, dictate as much of the report as she can, shut off the recorder, then go back to sleep.

For intense events from the past, things are more complicated. In some cases, if the experience isn't buried too deep, you can dictate the memory into a voice recorder, erase it, dictate it again, erase it, and do the whole thing all over again. "Verbalizing gets the memory out of storage, where you can deal with it so it won't come out and bother you during the night," says Dr. Yan-Go.

If that doesn't work, then you need to go into talk therapy and face the event before it will stop waking you up. "Denial is good when you're in Iraq and you have shrapnel in your shoulder," says the psychiatrist. "When you're drinking and thinking and not sleeping, it's bad.

"The bottom line is that we all have challenges in our lives. Some we can control; others we can't. What we can always change, however, is how we respond."

THE BIG SNORT

Until recently, sleep apnea—technically defined as pausing more than 10 seconds between breaths while you're sleeping—was thought to occur only in men.

More recently, however, researchers have found that it occurs in small numbers of younger women and that the risk increases with age. By menopause between 20 and 55 percent of women will have it. The condition will leave them snorting, snoring, and gasping for air by night, and exhausted, cranky, and headachy by day.

To hear what sleep apnea sounds like, go to www.sleep.rd.com. Then check out page 186 for tips on how to cope with this condition.

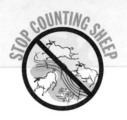

Sleep Like a Baby

Several nights a week more than half of us between the ages of 35 and 55 can't sleep. Here's how to turn that around.

THINK ABOUT SHORT-TERM HRT. Surprised? Hormone replacement therapy (HRT) has largely fallen out of favor among women and their doctors, and for good reason. Long-term research studies have found it can increase your risk of blood clots, breast cancer, and gallbladder disease.

Still, the fact is that perimenopausal women who use HRT sleep better. Whether it's because it reduces hot flushes or has some other effect isn't known.

How do you weigh the risks and benefits? "The risks and benefits of any treatment need to be individualized to your particular body—not just what the research says or professional scientific associations prescribe," says Becky Wang-Cheng, M.D., a medical director at Kettering Medical Center and author of *Menopause.*

If breast cancer runs in your family but hot flashes are preventing you from getting enough sleep to do your job, a super-low dose of hormones might be helpful despite the research. And we're not talking about long-term or daily use. "Sometimes just one pill a week is enough to keep symptoms in check," says Dr. Wang-Cheng.

JoAnn Manson, M.D., the Harvard researcher who pioneered much of the research that uncovered the dangers of HRT and author of *Hot Flashes, Hormones and Your Health*, agrees that HRT should still be an option for some women.

Most women do not need hormone therapy to get through the hormonal transition into menopause, says Dr. Manson. Menopause is natural, and we need to guard against the over-medicalization of our lives. "However, for about one in every five women, menopausal symptoms are severe enough to disrupt sleep and quality of life," she adds. "Hormone therapy still has an important role to play for such women."

REINFORCE YOUR SLEEP SCHEDULE. Like other kinds of insomnia, the sleeplessness of perimenopause can be overcome by sticking to the cycles of sleeping and waking that you have previously established with your biological clock. This helps your body override some of the conflicting messages it may be getting from wayward hormones activated by perimenopause.

It's important that you keep your sleeping and waking schedules pretty steady—no Sunday sleep-ins, for example—if you want to be able to count on good, restorative sleep during this uneasy stage of life. And good, restorative sleep is the best gift you can give yourself at this time.

If you don't already have a firm sleeping schedule, now is certainly the time to develop one. It isn't hard to do, and the benefits will serve you for the rest of your life.

CONSIDER AN ALTERNATIVE. Women who are reluctant to use estrogen may want to talk with their doctors about the antidepressant Effexor, says Dr. Wang-Cheng. It decreases the hot flushes that can disrupt sleep and is even prescribed by doctors for breast cancer patients who are undergoing active therapy.

"It's not as good as estrogen," adds the physician, "but it reduces hot flushes by 40 to 60 percent and will make you drowsy."

WORK WITH A THERAPIST. Eight or 10 weeks with a certified cognitive behavioral therapist will frequently give you a handful of sleep strategies custom-tailored to your particular issues during this life stage. If you're regularly waking up in the middle of the night and can't get back to sleep, however, you might find it more helpful to contact a psychiatrist to talk over old struggles that may be troubling you.

TAKE A SLEEP BREAK. After those nights when your reproductive hormones and the hormones that control your sleep/wake cycle really can't work together, try to get back some of the sleep you've lost by 4:00 P.M., says Dr. Yan-Go. Not all of it—that's not practical for most of us. Just take the edge off your drowsiness and you'll be surprised at how effectively your brain cells will start firing again. If you drive to work, go out to the car at lunch, put down the backseat, and snooze for 10 minutes. Or just put your head down on your desk for 5.

"I do that all the time," adds the psychiatrist. "People with sleep deprivation can go crazy!"

WICK AWAY THE PROBLEM. If hot flushes are your particular sleep disrupter, buy long johns, or gym shorts and T-shirts made from fabrics that athletes use to wick away moisture such as PowerDry and CoolMax. Then wear them as pj's. They won't stop a hot flush, but they'll keep it from turning into a majorly disruptive night sweat in which you have to get up and change clothes.

CHILL IN BED. Chillow is a pillow with a cooling water insert that lowers your body temperature. It won't stop hot flushes, but it can reduce their intensity and their ability to disrupt your sleep.

DROP YOUR TEMP. Lower the temperature of your bedroom before you climb into bed, says Dr. Wang-Cheng. Lower temperatures signal your body that it's time to sleep, and they make hot flushes less disruptive. If your bed partner objects, just tell him to bundle up.

A hot bath also helps you lower your body's temperature. Yeah, your temperature goes up while you're in the bath, but your body's response to the heat will be to drop your temperature.

As long as perimenopausal dryness hasn't resulted in painful intercourse, enjoy a quickie, suggests Dr. Wang-Cheng. Some 44 percent of perimenopausal women say they don't have time for sex. But the Big O is still one of the most sleep-inducing agents around. Just don't forget to protect yourself against an unanticipated side effect that could appear nine months later. Now that would *really* trash your sleep!

TONE IT DOWN. Toning down a jumpy sympathetic nervous system will encourage a balanced sleep/wake cycle in perimenopausal women, says Dr. Yan-Go. Think about tai chi, meditation, prayer, biofeedback, yoga—any activity that allows you to cultivate a peaceful center and a sense of balance.

If you enroll in a class for one of these, just keep one thing in mind. "Don't try to be perfect at it," says Dr. Yan-Go. "I tried tai chi, but kept wobbling when I had to stand on one foot." She kept trying to master the movements but ended up tying herself in knots—which is about as far from cultivating a peaceful center as she could get.

"Now I do yoga, where I can sit on my butt and not worry," chuckles the psychiatrist.

TALK TO A SLEEP DOC. If you suspect you have a sleep disorder involving breathing difficulties, restless legs, or narcolepsy, ask your primary-care physician for a referral to a sleep center for testing, diagnosis, and treatment. If your doctor doesn't know of one in the vicinity, flip to page 214. Chances are, we do.

Before and after Baby

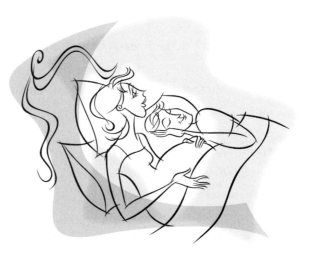

Ninety-seven percent of expectant moms report that they don't sleep in the third trimester. Forty-two percent of new moms claim they don't sleep.

> One-third of all pregnant women rarely or **never get a good night's sleep.**

What does that tell you?

In utero, out of utero, it doesn't really matter. A baby's sole purpose in life is to give you sweet smiles, right? Well, that may be true in our dreams. But the reality is dirty diapers, demanding cries, and the inability to close your eyes for 10 minutes straight.

All is not lost, however. Here's how you can beat pregnancy insomnia and then outfox those new little critters with the 31 mother-tested tips in this section.

Pregnancy Insomnia: Sleeping for Two

Thirty-four-year-old Becky Hanf Nezin experiences pregnancy the way every woman wishes she could. She sleeps like a log at night, wakes up refreshed in the morning, and stays in shape by running after her five kids and walking along country roads near her home in Lincoln, Vermont.

"All of my pregnancies were uneventful," says Becky, long blond hair swinging over her shoulder as she lifts Adeline, her three-month-old daughter, for a cuddle.

"But I was exhausted every day at about 2:30," she adds ruefully. "Right when the kids came home from school."

Less Sleep = More Labor

Except for that one little glitch, Becky was fortunate. Some 80 percent of women in their first trimester report that they have trouble sleeping, and a whopping 97 percent are tossing and turning by their third.

That's serious stuff. Aside from the fact that a lot of cellular growth and system repair takes place at night and that without a good night's sleep most of us are pretty miserable people, a study at the University of California, San Francisco, found that women who averaged less than 6 hours of sleep a night had 10 hours more labor than women who got

Help Me! I'm Up!

Go into the room you're preparing for the baby. Click on the night-light, sit in the rocker, and pull a warm shawl around your shoulders. Slip your arms around your growing belly and rock your baby. Then return to your bed, close your eyes, and think of the new life stirring within.

7 or more hours of sleep. And women who slept under 6 hours a night were more than *four* times more likely to require a cesarean delivery.

So what's going on?

"Sleep changes in a couple of different ways during pregnancy," explains Grace Pien, M.D., a sleep researcher at the University of Pennsylvania's Center for Sleep and Respiratory Neurobiology. "Women often say that they get a lot sleepier just a few weeks after they become pregnant. But they also find that even if they're sleeping seven or eight hours a night, they're still tired during the day."

The sleepiness seems to be caused by the first-trimester rise in hormones, says Dr. Pien. Practically from the moment of conception, progesterone floods your body to support the pregnancy, bringing with it the sometimes overwhelming need to sleep at any time and any place. It also tends to make you nauseous, increase your body temperature, and tweak your urinary tract muscles so you're heading off to the bathroom every 10 minutes. So even though the progesterone encourages you to spend time in bed, the sleep you get is often fragmented and less than restorative.

Who's Up?

80 percent of women in their first trimester, 97 percent of women in their third trimester, and any guy married to them.

The second trimester is better, says Dr. Pien. Women have more energy, and they feel more alert. The fetus moves higher in the abdomen, which reduces pressure on the bladder and the need to stay close to a bathroom. But sleep is beginning to get lighter, there's less restorative deep sleep, and the physical discomfort is growing.

By the third trimester women are frequently experiencing heartburn, backaches, and breathlessness as the growing fetus displaces their stomach and diaphragm and reaches maximum weight. What's more, some 75 percent of women experience leg cramps, 20 percent experience restless legs syndrome outright (see "Kick the Restless Legs" on page 184), and absolutely nobody can find a comfortable position in which to sleep.

Not that anyone's sleeping. Those frequent visits to the bathroom are back. In spades.

One Woman's Story

Vancouver mom Karen Norvell, 39, loves kids. She has two herself, and she offers child care to neighborhood moms. But as much as she loves children, Karen has no intention of ever getting pregnant again.

"I've had restless legs syndrome since I was in my teens," Karen explains. "I'd always get a sensation in my legs before my period—a funny feeling that made me want to move them. I'd have a bad night with no sleep, I'd feel bloated and cranky, and I'd have to keep moving my legs."

Karen sighs. "I always thought it was part of 'that time of the month,' until it got more severe when I was pregnant. I ended up at my doctor's office in tears." Nothing could keep her legs still. Warm baths didn't work; relaxation exercises were a joke. The minute she'd lie down, the tingles and twitches would start up.

Once she started nursing, however, the urge to move her legs stopped. But as soon as she started menstruating again, the tingles and twitches were back. Fortunately, "it went back to being just a couple of nights a month, right before my period," says Karen. "And that I could manage."

Then she got pregnant again. "I couldn't take sleeping pills because of the baby, so my doctor suggested a bit of wine every night. It worked for a couple of weeks."

Eventually, Karen outran the problem. "I started staying up at night and sleeping in the day," she explains. Then after a couple of weeks, as soon as I'd lie down during the day, it would start up." At her wit's end, she kept moving day and night, falling asleep in front of the TV or wherever she could to catch a few hours' sleep. She'd feel the tingle and have to leap up.

It wasn't an experience she cares to repeat. "You start thinking funny when you don't sleep for a few weeks," she comments wryly.

"I'd love more kids, but I just can't do it."

THE BIG SNORE

Between increased progesterone and increased physical discomfort, you'd think that pregnant women had enough on their plates. But as many a husband can attest, even the quietest woman can snore with the best of the log-sawers when she's pregnant.

Studies show that about 4 percent of women snore *before* they get pregnant, but by the *end* of their pregnancies, 25 percent of women snore occasionally and *another* 25 percent snore loudly.

The propensity to snore is apparently caused by a woman's own increasing estrogen. The hormone causes capillaries throughout the body to swell—which gives pregnant women that "puffy" look. Unfortunately, when nose capillaries swell, they can partially block nasal passages. Hence the snoring.

All snoring is a pain, for both you and your bed partner. But there's a difference between snoring that simply disrupts your partner's sleep and snoring that signals a more serious problem for you and your baby, says Grace Pien, M.D., a researcher at the University of Pennsylvania's Center for Sleep and Respiratory Neurobiology.

"If your husband says, 'Honey, you started snoring,' that's probably not going to be worrisome," she says. "But if he says, `Honey, you started snoring and I wasn't sure if you were breathing last night,' then you should talk to your doctor—and consider going to a sleep center for a sleep study."

The problem is that you might be developing sleep apnea, a condition in which you can literally stop breathing for several seconds up to a hundred times a night. (For more information see page 186.) You may not even be aware of it since your brain will eventually wake you up to grab that next breath, but your sleep will be far from restful and you'll wake headachy and groggy in the morning.

"Snoring is something we don't entirely understand," says Dr. Pien, who has studied disordered breathing in pregnant women. "We don't know if it's harmful."

In nonpregnant women the obstructed breathing of sleep apnea will put women at risk of heart disease and a shorter lifespan.

In pregnant women the concern is that obstructed breathing may reduce the amount of oxygen available to the fetus, or it may trigger high blood pressure or preeclampsia in the mother. There's even the possibility that preeclampsia or high blood pressure triggers snoring.

In a small study of 100 pregnant women conducted by Dr. Pien, so far that doesn't seem to be the case. "We found that women who developed mild sleep-disordered breathing did not appear to be at increased risk for preeclampsia or high blood pressure," says Dr. Pien. "So if you develop sleep apnea during pregnancy, it looks as though it may not be harmful to either you or your baby."

But that's mild snoring and mild sleep apnea, she cautions. Women with a Body Mass Index over 30, women who were diagnosed with sleep apnea before pregnancy, women who develop *severe* sleep apnea during pregnancy, and women whose oxygen levels, as measured by their doctors, fall significantly in pregnancy could get into serious trouble. So women in each of these groups should be evaluated at a sleep center.

Fortunately, sleep apnea can be treated by a pressurized nighttime supply of oxygen that keeps the airway open.

When Is Snoring Dangerous to Your Pregnancy?

- When you snore loudly with brief pauses in which you're not breathing

- When you have a Body Mass Index over 30

- When you've been diagnosed with sleep apnea prior to pregnancy

- When you have low oxygen levels, as measured by your doctor

Beating Pregnancy Insomnia

Okay. So you're tossing and turning, snoring and snorting, aching, kicking, getting up to go to the bathroom, and trying every which way to find a comfortable position. It's not easy to sleep through the middle of all that—and some nights it seems downright hopeless. But here's what will give you the best chance.

SKIP THE NAPS. Daytime sleepiness, particularly in the first trimester, encourages almost every pregnant woman to nap. But naps make it more difficult to sleep at night because they take away some of the sleep pressure that builds up over the day.

"It's like snacking," says Grace Pien, M.D., a sleep researcher at the University of Pennsylvania's Center for Sleep and Respiratory Neurobiology. "Eating even a small amount of food before a meal can take away your appetite."

CANCEL THE SLEEP DEBT. Most women sleep only 6½ hours a night, so they head into pregnancy with a sleep debt. Fortunately, it's possible to repay that debt and bring your body back into balance before pregnancy makes sleeping harder.

To avoid napping, try going to bed an hour earlier than usual on a regular basis. If 11 o'clock is your usual time, head into the bedroom at 10. So maybe you'll miss your favorite TV show or that report you were working on just won't get done. Just keep in mind the University of California, San Francisco (UCSF), study that found that a woman who sleeps less than 6 hours a night quadruples her risk of a C-section and can add up to 10 hours to her labor. That's a great incentive to end the day early.

ADDRESS ANXIETY; BUFFER STRESS. Both anxiety and stress have very real physiological components, says sleep researcher Kathryn Lee, Ph.D., the UCSF professor who uncovered the relationship between poor sleep and length and complications of labor. In fact, she's betting that it was anxiety and stress that kept the women in her study from sleeping and, ultimately, led to increased labor and a complicated delivery.

"When you're exhausted, your muscles are tired," explains Dr. Lee. So if women are losing sleep because they're worrying about the baby, or anxious about their new roles, or anxious about how they're going to earn a living, or any one of the million and one things that run through an about-to-be mom's head at 2 in the morning, it's likely that the women were going into labor with tired muscles. "And if those muscles were tired, there's a good chance they might not have been pushing as well as they needed to," she says.

Talk to friends and family about any concerns that are keeping you up at night, or schedule a few quick visits to a therapist who can help you address the anxiety they may be generating. And learn how to use prayer, yoga, or meditation to connect with the calming stillness that lies at the very center of each and every one of us. The fruits of your efforts may be a shorter and safer labor.

BUY LOTS OF PILLOWS. No matter how you lie, you'll need lots of support to get comfortable by the third trimester. Start with a full-length body pillow, then add smaller pillows for extra support. Some women like pillows under their heads and under their arms; others also like them stuffed between baby belly and bed, wedged between knees, and snuggled into the small of their backs. Suit yourself.

DON'T SWEAT THE DREAMS. A Canadian study recently revealed that 59 percent of pregnant women have horrific dreams that their baby is in some kind of danger. The dreams are normal, apparently part of a woman's instinct to protect her child. If one wakes you up, don't think it's a premonition. Just roll over and go back to sleep.

WARM THE LAVENDER. Some pillows come microwave-safe and scented with natural lavender. Follow package directions for heating, then lie down, tuck the pillow wherever you ache, close your eyes, and relax into the warm scent. You'll be asleep in no time.

HOLD THE LIQUID AFTER 4:00 P.M. As any potty-training mom knows, you fill your kid full of water and juice all day long until around 4 o'clock. Then you give him liquids only when he asks for them, and then in quarter-cup amounts. As a result, your kid can sleep through the night and wake up dry, rested, and proud the next day.

The same thing works with pregnant moms, says Dr. Pien. Some of those nighttime trips are due to your physiology. But there's also another reason: Most pregnant women are busy all day long and don't take time to drink and stay hydrated. So when they get home, they tend to tank up. The fact that they need to get up and urinate during the night is a natural consequence. A better approach is to carry a large water bottle with you all day—and finish it before you leave work.

REMEMBER MAMA. When your mom's back ached, she likely reached for a heating pad and put it on her hips. You should do the same. Just keep it set on low, and don't fall asleep while it's on.

GET OUT THE BATH TOYS. Slide into a tub of warm water before bed and splash around, suggests Dr. Pien. Avoid hot water since some studies indicate that it can cause vasoconstriction, which can lead to miscarriage.

KEEP A REGULAR SLEEP SCHEDULE. Yes, even on weekends. Your body uses light to regulate its sleep/wake cycle. If it gets confused, you could be tossing and turning for hours.

DEAL WITH NAUSEA. Munch on a few crackers several times during the day. Daytime munching seems to head off nighttime nausea.

BAG THE FRIED FOOD. Also, spicy or acidic anything. Heartburn at 3:00 A.M. is not a good life choice.

EAT SMALL. Several small, light meals during the day instead of a heavier one at night will encourage deeper sleep.

KICK BUTTS. Say yes the next time someone asks, "Mind if I smoke?" A study of more than 35,000 pregnant women conducted at Nihon University in Tokyo found that women exposed to secondhand tobacco smoke were more likely to have trouble falling asleep and staying asleep than women who weren't. They also had breathing difficulties and were more likely to awake at the crack of dawn.

WORK OUT. A 30-minute daily workout will strengthen your body and get you in shape for labor and delivery. Brisk walking, lap swimming, stationary or recumbent biking, and a low-impact aerobics class designed for pregnant women are best. Check with your doctor before you start.

If you haven't been exercising regularly, begin slowly, say, 5 minutes a day. Add 5 minutes a week until you're up to 30 minutes a day. Avoid exercising in hot weather, and after the first trimester avoid doing exercises while lying on your back. Otherwise, you go, girl!

BASK IN THE SUN. A little natural-light exposure during the afternoon will help your body clock understand when you're supposed to be awake—and when you're supposed to be asleep.

KEEP THE PARENTING BOOKS IN THE LIVING ROOM. If you read parenting books right before you turn out the light, chances are you'll be running if-then and what-if scenarios in your head for hours to come. This is daytime work.

PUT AWAY THE PAINT CHIPS AND CATALOGS. Okay, we know you love poring over paint chips and baby furniture catalogs and making plans for the nursery. But right before bed? Isn't that a little stimulating?

STRIP THE BEDROOM. "The bedroom is for sleep and sex," says Dr. Pien, repeating the mantra of sleep medicine specialists everywhere. Remove the TV, computer, Palm Pilot, cell phone, and anything else that's unrelated to those two most pleasurable activities.

Postpartum Insomnia: Planning Your Strategy

There is no way that a new mother can get a good night's sleep. Her hormones are crashing, her pelvis is battered, the baby is crying, her mother's moved in for the duration, and her mother-in-law wants to know why she named the baby Emma.

TOO BLUE

Postpartum blues, which occur three to five days after birth, are a natural consequence of hormonal changes and, possibly, insomnia during the last trimester.

They last roughly a week. If they last longer, keep an eye out for the following symptoms since you may be heading into postpartum depression, a serious mood disorder that requires treatment. Sometimes simply more help with the baby and more time for yourself will help, but other times antidepressants may be necessary. Call your doctor immediately if these symptoms seem to be emerging:

- Increased crying

- Unexplained weight changes

- Restlessness

- Irritability

- Anxiety

- Feeling guilty

- Feeling that life's not worth living

- No appetite

- Lack of pleasure in formerly pleasurable activities

- Sleeping more

- Unable to get to sleep

- Unable to stay asleep

- Little energy

- Having thoughts of hurting yourself

- Worrying about hurting your baby

Sleep? Not on your life. At least, not through the whole night. A reported 42 percent of new moms never get a good night's sleep. If you're up, 10 to 1 it's because your baby is up. And if you've already fed and changed the little lamb chop, try any of the following:

- Snuggle the baby close to your body.
- Encourage sucking—finger, breast, or pacifier is good.
- Rock—and rock and rock....
- Massage the baby lightly with an organic vegetable oil.
- Wake up the baby's father and hand her over.

"I close my eyes, and I make up a story with a happy ending based on real people, places, and things in my life. I rarely get to finish the story, but it feels good getting there."
—JULIE EVANS

Who's Up?

74 percent of moms who stay at home, 54 percent of moms who work full-time outside the home, and 16 percent of moms who work part-time

Around 50 percent of babies sleep through the night at two months, 75 percent at three months. Other factors that disrupt a new mother's sleep are stress, role expectations, family support, and one or two politically correct but slightly quirky child-care trends that have evolved in recent years.

Quirkiness notwithstanding, every new mother *can* cobble together a plan to get the rest she needs. It just takes planning.

"With each new baby, my insomnia grew. 'New mom' took a backseat to chauffeur, laundress, and reading, writing, and arithmetic tutor. I was cranky all day long. Finally, I decided to change my bedtime to 8:00 P.M.—after nursing my daughter. At midnight I'd wake again for another feeding but would stay up to accomplish one of the things on my to-do list. Once done, I went back to bed feeling a little more comforted knowing I was ahead of the game even before the sun rose—and had freed myself up for a nap the next day."
—BARBARA BOOTH

Your New Baby Sleep Strategy

As fatigued as you may feel, start figuring out how you'll deal with sleep issues while you're still in the third trimester. Here's what we mean.

RECOGNIZE THE IMPORTANCE OF SLEEP. Sometimes it seems as though our culture has begun to view sleep as a sign of weakness. It's the new macho—and women are buying into it big-time.

"I can stay awake through anything."

"I can stay awake longer than you can."

"I can run on dead brain cells, sheer guts, and sheep entrails."

That's the kind of talk you often hear in the latte line at Starbucks. But your body was programmed to spend one-third of its life asleep, and to sleep in specific cycles of light sleep, deep sleep, and active-brain sleep. Each cycle takes 90 minutes, and each has a specific assignment that affects thinking, memory, growth, your immune system, and even your weight. Trying to tuck anything that important into an hour here and an hour there just won't get the job done. Especially not when you're also trying to nurture a new life.

SCHEDULE A DRESS REHEARSAL. "Starting during the last trimester, have your partner get out of work an hour early and pick up dinner on the way home," says Kathryn Lee, Ph.D., a sleep researcher at the University of California, San Francisco. "It sounds simple, but in our culture most guys haven't had the responsibility of thinking about what's for dinner, shopping for the ingredients, and delivering it to the table." The practice not only smoothes things out, she adds, it also gives you a break toward the end of pregnancy, when you're most likely to be exhausted and in need of a nap.

INVESTIGATE WORK OPTIONS. "Most women today are getting the message that they can do it all," says Dr. Lee. "And they can. They can be a mother really well, and do their job really well, and juggle everything."

"In fact," she says, chuckling, "I think there's some gene in there that allows women to multitask."

That's not to say that women shouldn't try to strike some kind of reasonable balance between work and family, adds Dr. Lee. Especially if they want some sleep. A poll for the National Sleep Foundation found that women who work full-time and have kids got the least sleep of all moms surveyed. Some 54 percent said they frequently woke during the night, and 56 percent said they often woke up feeling unrefreshed. Most kept going by downing caffeinated beverages and by giving up sleep (60 percent), exercise (60 percent), time with family and friends (52 percent), leisure activities (49 percent), and sex (44 percent).

Their partners must be thrilled.

But women who stay at home with their kids also don't sleep too well, according to the survey. A whopping 74 percent said they frequently had insomnia. Researchers suspect that it's because they don't set their body's internal clock by getting up at the same time every morning as would someone who had to be at her desk at a particular time.

Only mothers who work part-time seem to have it all together. A relatively small, 16 percent reported a sleep problem. The other 84 percent seemed to be doing just fine.

FOLLOW YOUR BODY'S NATURAL RHYTHMS. When deciding who's going to get up with the baby at night, keep in mind your natural programming, says Dr. Lee. "Your body is hormonally programmed to wake up at the least little gurgle, and the hormone prolactin causes your breasts to fill up and get uncomfortable just about the time the baby gets hungry." That doesn't mean you have to be on call 24/7, she adds, but it's something you need to factor into your decision.

LET DAD PINCH-HIT. One option is to put the baby to bed at night after the 8 o'clock feeding and go to bed yourself. Your partner can use a bottle of expressed milk to feed the baby around 10. Afterward your partner can go to bed and you can get up for the 2 to 4 feeding. That way, each of you will have the opportunity to have an uninterrupted six-plus hours of sleep.

MEND FAMILY FEUDS. You're going to need every hand on board if you plan on getting any sleep. In other cultures, grandparents are much more involved with new babies than they are in the United States, says Dr. Lee.

But there's no reason why it has to be that way. Especially if you have other children, why not ask one set of grandparents to come and help for a couple of weeks after the baby's born? Ask the other set to come for the following two weeks. Heck, invite any unencumbered aunts and uncles to come lend a hand as well—for a short time. Just make it clear to everyone that they're coming to make dinner, wash dishes, change diapers, give baths, and clean the house. An hour cuddling your baby is their reward. Plus, of course, a happy, well-rested new mom.

SLEEP WHEN BABY SLEEPS. A new baby will sleep 16 to 17 hours a day for a maximum of 4 to 5 hours at a time, pediatricians say. Once awake, a newborn will stay awake for only 1 to 2 hours max. Sleep while you can. Put your head down when your baby goes down. You might actually get a full cycle of sleep a couple of times a day.

UNPLUG THE PHONE. Aside from food, the most important thing to your health and the health of your baby may well be sleep. It affects your ability to function—to think, remember, heal, and take action— while it affects your baby's ability to grow physically and mentally. Sleep is sacred. Naps—both the baby's naps every couple of hours or yours, also hopefully every couple of hours—should not be disrupted just because someone outside the house has decided he or she needs to talk with you.

LEAVE DAD IN BED. Since it's usually Dad who gets up and goes off to work in the early weeks while Mom is on maternity leave, why not leave Dad in bed when the baby gets up during the night and have him come home an hour early from work to take responsibility for baby and dinner, suggests Dr. Lee. Not having to think about what to make for dinner, or make sure the groceries are in the kitchen, or actually prepare the meal is a nice chunk of time that you can use to shower, nap, or otherwise nurture yourself later in the day.

If Dad doesn't feel like making dinner, says Dr. Lee, he can pick up an extra quart of soup from the company cafeteria at noon and stick it in the office fridge until he goes home. Or he can bring home a roasted chicken and some veggies and a container of fresh fruit from the neighborhood market. Or he can pick up Chinese. Whatever. The point is that *you* don't have to think about it, shop for it, or make it.

DISCOURAGE VISITORS. Everybody wants to see the new baby, of course. And you, you conscientious person, will feel the need to make sure the house is clean and there's something to offer them when they come—your home-baked pound cake, some sandwiches, a little coffee, and maybe some tea, right?

Wrong. Unless your family has moved in to take over such chores, ask visitors to hold off for a week or so, then have them come one or two at a time for only an hour a couple of days a week. Anyone who's had kids will understand, and those who haven't will learn soon enough.

IGNORE FADS. Whatever you do, don't try to be politically correct at the expense of common sense. "I don't know how this all started, but there's this trend here in California where a husband and wife do this kind of contract with each other before the baby is born," says Dr. Lee. "The contract is that the father will get up during the night and bring the baby to the mother so that she can breastfeed. Afterward he changes the baby and everyone goes back to sleep.

"I guess it's one way of thinking that everybody's participating in child care," says Dr. Lee, "but what it means is that nobody's sleeping and everybody's tired.

"It could make sense in some families," she adds, "but to me it means that none of the adults is sleeping. That means that no one is able to make a coherent decision—and that sounds really dangerous."

SLEEP TOGETHER. In the past, studies have linked the practice of sleeping with your baby to maternal insomnia. But in many of these studies, a mother's insomnia was caused mainly by her fear that the baby would be smothered by the sheets, roll out of bed, or be rolled upon by one of the parents.

In a soon-to-be-released study of 140 couples and their babies, Dr. Lee has discovered that moms actually sleep better when the baby sleeps in a bassinette next to the parents' bed rather than in his or her own room down the hall.

"The idea is that the baby's within easy reach, the mother doesn't have to be aroused by the baby's screaming, and she doesn't have to get up, turn on the lights, and go down a hallway," says Dr. Lee. That makes it easier to slide back into sleep after the feeding.

The trick is to put a white-noise machine and a night-light at the foot of the bed, says Dr. Lee. The night-light allows the mother to check on her child without rousing both of them with bright lights, and the machine masks the little noises that babies always make, so they don't disturb the mother—particularly in her hormone-influenced hyperalert state. It's only when the baby starts to fuss that the mother is actually awakened. The baby doesn't have to work him- or herself into a window-rattling cry to get fed, so mom is less aroused. What's more, it turns out that babies like this little routine, too. Dr. Lee's data show that babies seem to slide back into sleep much easier as well.

What's more, the white-noise machine filters out Daddy's snoring—a little extra benefit.

EXPECT THE BLUES. When all those hormones surging through your body to help maintain your pregnancy are suddenly shut off at birth, your body's going to react. In fact, in some cases it almost seems akin to drug withdrawal. Possibly as a consequence, some 35 to 80 percent of women get the blues, which start three to five days after birth and last roughly a week.

Unfortunately, somewhere around 10 percent of new moms will actually tumble into a postpartum depression that begins somewhere between the second and fourth week. The difference between the blues and postpartum depression? It seems to be a question of degree—and only a doctor should judge the difference.

No one knows what causes postpartum depression. Some researchers think it's the postpartum drop in hormones, but then why don't we all get it? Other researchers feel it's a lack of support at home, and a few think it occurs because society "expects" us to be depressed. And some, perhaps mothers themselves, feel that researchers should try to toss and turn for the last three months of pregnancy as most women do, experience 15 hours of labor, then top it all off by having to wake up three times a night for the next three months and see how happy and even-tempered they are.

In fact, there are now a couple of studies that are beginning to support precisely that notion.

FIND YOUR BABY'S RHYTHM. Pediatricians tell us that up until three or four months of age, a baby's sleep is determined purely and simply by its biological needs, and the best thing for both you and the baby is to simply roll with those needs. Your baby will grow and you'll get a good night's sleep.

Eventually.

Sleep Eating

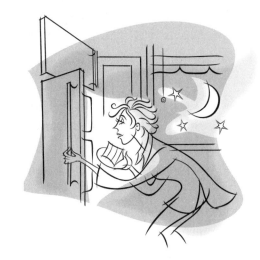

Food as a sleep saboteur?

Absolutely. And we aren't talking about nights when you try the new sushi place down the street and end up with dancing shrimp doing the rumba through your gut.

Instead, we're talking about a saboteur called sleep-related eating disorder (SRED). Also called nocturnal binge-eating disorder, it's a condition in which eating during the middle of the night is likely to keep you from getting the deep restorative sleep you need—and it may force you to gain serious amounts of weight.

> Sometimes the only clue to a sleep-eating problem is a trail of bread crumbs.

The disorder affects more than 4 percent of young adults, researchers report, and triple that number among those who have been diagnosed with eating disorders such as anorexia or bulimia. It may go on undetected for a whopping 10 years before weight gain, high blood sugar, high cholesterol, major depression, and disrupted sleep reveal its presence to a physician's discerning eye.

Out of Control

Sometimes the only clue you have to SRED is the trail of bread crumbs you leave behind. You wake up on the groggy side, feeling stuffed and a little anorexic, walk to the kitchen, and there you find the remnants of a midnight snack—usually high-fat, high-calorie foods. There are probably no fruits or vegetables, but there may well be such oddities as buttered cigarettes, dog food, salt sandwiches, even eggshells, and—dangerously—kitchen cleaners.

The out-of-control eating occurs almost nightly, sometimes more than once a night. It begins after a period of sleep. The next morning the sleep eater may be able to recall vague images of what she did. Or not.

Scientists are just beginning to unravel the complicated brain circuitry that connects eating and sleeping. But they have been able to figure out that SRED is sometimes associated with sleep disorders such as restless legs, narcolepsy, or obstructive sleep apnea and can be triggered by medications such as zolpidem (Ambien), triazolam (Halcion), and lithium (Lithobid). It can also apparently be triggered by major relationship stress, by dieting, and by the cessation of cigarette smoking, alcohol, and recreational drugs.

EATING DISORDERS SABOTAGE SLEEP

Both anorexia nervosa, a disorder in which (mostly) women eat between 400 and 800 calories a day, and bulimia nervosa, a disorder in which (mostly) women eat between 10,000 and 30,000 calories a day, significantly interfere with sleep. Because those with anorexia frequently use the time they would normally sleep to exercise, and those with bulimia frequently stay up all night eating, neither of the groups function on the recommended amount of sleep.

One Woman's Story

When 36-year-old Molly Johnson's husband began waking her up on a regular basis to ask about bills she hadn't paid or chores she hadn't done during the day, she couldn't believe it.

"I'm a strong person by nature," says Molly, an elementary school substitute teacher, "but I couldn't handle the stress. I became riddled with anxiety. And I began to dread the night because I didn't know if it was going to be a good one or not."

Eventually, she says, her husband's behavior not only disrupted her sleep when he woke her, her fear that he might wake her kept her from sleeping as well.

She's not sure exactly when it was that she started waking up in the middle of the night to eat, but eventually she would wake twice a night and head for the kitchen to eat chips, cookies, candy, and just about anything that wasn't nailed down. She wasn't asleep exactly, but she wasn't awake, either. "I knew what I was doing," she says, "but in a sleepy, dreamlike way."

Molly tried therapy for four years, and finally, at her psychiatrist's urging, she went on an antidepressant. The drug made her less anxious, she says, but neither the therapy nor the antidepressant helped with her sleep eating.

Then one day she decided that she was going to spend the night in her daughter's bedroom, thinking that her husband wouldn't wake her if her daughter was present. It worked. Her husband's intrusive behavior came to a halt—and so did her sleep eating.

Today she sleeps well. "Sleeping in separate bedrooms has saved me," she says. "I traded intimacy and sex for solace and peace."

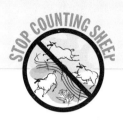

Stop Sabotaging Your Sleep

SRED, or sleep-related eating disorder, is a serious problem. It not only can make you gain serious amounts of weight and disrupt your sleep, it may also cause you to inadvertently eat toxic substances or foods to which you're allergic. Here's how to get a handle on it.

SEE YOUR DOCTOR. If you're gaining weight and discovering a mess in the kitchen every morning, talk to your doctor about whether or not you might have SRED. Tell her about any medications you're taking that she might not know about, including any recreational drugs or alcohol. Tell her about your eating habits, relationships, and any recent dieting. Even if she can't find the precise cause of your eating, there are medications she can prescribe that will help you control the disorder.

STAY OFF DIETS. Dieting is a natural response to the weight gain you're experiencing, but it may be counterproductive. In fact, it may be exacerbating your problem. Run any low-calorie eating plans by your doctor.

REBUILD RELATIONSHIPS. If a close relationship with a parent or partner is stressing you out, see a therapist pronto. You could be paying the price of a nonfunctional relationship with your health.

FRISK YOUR HOME. Get everything out of your home that would be harmful if you ate it. That means kitchen cleaners, bathroom cleaners, paint, lamp oil, whatever. Leave medication at the office or with a trusted friend—anywhere you can get it when you need it, but not at home while you're sleep eating.

Dealing with Illness

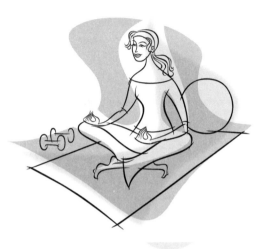

Three of the most constant impediments to sleep are allergies, cancer, and pain. Any one of them can keep you from getting to sleep, keep you from settling into a restorative sleep, wake you throughout the night, or cause you to wake—and stay awake—

"Sleeping well will help you heal optimally," says Julie Silver, M.D.

just before dawn. And, of course, we need sleep to cope with the stress contributed by illness.

Fortunately, all three of these disruptive problems are manageable, and with the proper solution sleep is not only possible but can also contribute to fighting the underlying causes of each of these health issues. Soon you'll be feeling more positive, more well rested, and better equipped to deal with the days ahead.

Allergies

We stumble into our workplace each morning exhausted—with itchy, swollen faces, plugged-up noses, and big circles under our eyes—and try to do our jobs feeling as though we are sloughing through a mudslide on the California coast.

For some 50 million of us, it's an annual rite of spring. Or summer. Or fall. And winter, too, come to think of it.

The problem is our allergies. In spring our immune systems rev up to repel what they perceive as a life-threatening invader: tree pollen. If you're allergic to tree pollen and there's an oak, western red cedar, elm, birch, ash hickory, poplar, sycamore, maple, cypress, or walnut tree in the area, you're cooked. You will cough, sneeze, hack, and blow with the best of us.

In summer outdoor mold, weeds, and grasses add to the problem. Strange plants called *Alternaria*, *Cladosporium*, and *Aspergillus*—otherwise known as mold—send their spores into the air from the first spring thaw

WHY ME?

It's the luck o' the genes.

The genes your parents handed you at conception have interacted with something in the environment they just don't like. So they've decided to have a fit every time they see that substance entering your body, whether it is pollen or mold or something no one's even discovered yet.

Whatever the allergen is, your genes have programmed an army of defensive immune-system players to take it out. Unfortunately, in the truly heroic performance of their job, those immune-system players cause all the symptoms you have come to know and love: stuffy nose, postnasal drip, sneezes, itches, and so on.

to the first freeze in the northern and eastern United States, and all year long in the South and along the West Coast. Timothy, Bermuda, sweet vernal, red top, and blue grasses float their pollen after them. In fall it's ragweed pollen that stuffs your nose and prevents sleep—with a little help from sagebrush, pigweed, tumbleweed, Russian thistle, and cockleweed.

And since winter is when we are more likely to be shut up inside with dust mites, animal dander, and indoor molds, that's when some of us not only have allergies, but we develop what some have called "the sinuses from hell." Not only can't we breathe or sleep, we also get a massive headache when we lie down.

One Woman's Story

GLADYS WATTS: Sleepless in Vermont

When Vermont writer Gladys Watts heads for bed in fall, winter, and spring, she knows that allergies will wake her up in the middle of the night unless she takes a few precautions.

So although her husband hoots and hollers at the sight of his wife building a Mount Everest of pillows to keep her head elevated, she does what she has to do. She builds the mound, fills a sports water bottle and places it on the nightstand, then checks the contents of a Nantucket fisherman's basket she keeps beside it that holds her anti-allergy arsenal. After spritzing her nostrils with a saline nasal spray that contains eucalyptus along with the saline, she hops into bed.

"I'd rather do almost anything than not sleep," says Gladys. "My allergies make me groggy as it is. If I can't sleep as well,"—she shrugs her shoulders—"I'll be totally nonfunctional the next day. So I do anything I can to keep allergies under control at night."

Gladys is one of the thousands of women who are allergic to tree pollen. So during the spring—which in Vermont is more like late May

"Allergy can have a significant impact on our ability to enjoy a satisfying night's sleep," explains allergist William H. Anderson, M.D., a member of the American Academy of Allergy, Asthma, and Immunology who practices in Bellingham, Washington. "In fact, there will be some nights when you'll wake up in the middle of the night and feel as though someone had pinched your nose shut."

> "I always keep half a Benadryl on my night table and take it in the middle of the night if I wake up and can't get back to sleep. Works every time."
> —ALISON MUNOZ

and early June—she's careful to keep her bedroom windows closed as well as keep her anti-allergy arsenal stocked.

But she's also allergic to dust. And even though she vacuums and dusts the bedroom faithfully once a week, launders her sheets and comforter in hot water, uses synthetic window shades instead of curtains, and sleeps on an allergy-proof pillow, her dust allergies act up fall and winter. So for nine months out of the year, her mound of pillows and anti-allergy arsenal are the only thing that assures her of a good night's sleep.

At night when her nasal passages get stuffy, a postnasal drip makes her cough, or her sinuses start to throb, she turns on the tiny book light mounted on her basket and pulls out the saline spray. If that doesn't unclog things, she uses one squirt of a low-power nasal spray decongestant. That usually takes care of the problem.

But to delay the congestion from returning, she takes a tube of nasal cream with eucalyptus and rubs a tiny bit of it around the outside of her nostrils. And because her lips are chapped and her throat is dry from trying to breathe through her mouth, she sips a little water, then applies lip balm to her lips.

Then, snapping off her book light, Gladys Watts slips easily into a very deep, very restful sleep.

THE FAKE

Allergy symptoms can be triggered as a side effect of medications prescribed for high blood pressure or erectile dysfunction. Oral contraceptives can cause similar effects. There's no real allergy involved—just the symptoms. Check with your doctor if you suspect a medication might be causing *your* allergy.

Unfortunately, that means the allergen has triggered an inflammation of the mucous membrane lining the nasal passages. The lining swells and impedes the normal flow of air and oxygen into your lungs. You gasp, you choke, you cough—you do a lot of things, but none of them involve sleep.

Making things worse is the fact that a number of the chemicals your immune system produces in response to the allergen—histamine, leukotrienes, cytokines, and prostaglandins—not only play a role in closing down your airway, they also play a role in sleep regulation.

In other words, you are in a tough place. If the stuffy nose and sneezing don't get you, the immunomodulators (don't you just love that word?) will. And no one will be sleeping when they do.

"My yoga teacher recommended that I purchase a netti pot (a ceramic one because plastic can't be sanitized thoroughly) to relieve my allergy symptoms, and it has changed my life. I fill the pot with warm water and ½ teaspoon of non-iodized salt and then, while bending over a sink, I pour the water first into my right nostril and then the left. I follow this procedure both in the morning and at night. The theory is that the cilia in our nasal and sinus passages when cleansed on a regular basis become rejuvenated and improve their filtering capability. I never fail to feel less stuffy after I've used it. I'll never be without a netti pot again." —PAM DELSONNO

Prevent Allergy Sleep Loss

Not only does the sheer misery induced by allergy symptoms keep you awake at night, but your body's immunological response to those allergens disrupts the systems set up to regulate your sleep. So the key to a good night's sleep is to keep allergens at bay—or, when that's simply impossible, find a way to minimize your body's reaction to them. Here's how to do it.

MAKE A BATTLE PLAN. Get an ID on the allergens that are driving you crazy, find out when and how they appear, then formulate a battle plan with your doctor. Include everything from reducing contact with the allergen to treating it with medication.

If your allergies aren't immediately obvious to you and your doctor, ask your doctor for a referral to an allergist in your community. Or go to www.aaaai.org, click on "patients and consumers," then click on "find an allergist." Your allergist will run a series of skin or blood tests to reveal specific allergens.

WASH. When allergens, dust, and mold enter your nasal passages, they tend to get stuck in the membrane lining those passages. Inflammation sets in, your nose becomes swollen and clogged, and a nasty sinus infection can be the result.

Fortunately, however, "nasal irrigation, if it is done correctly and gently, can remove allergens, irritants, and inflammatory mucus," says William H. Anderson, M.D., a member of the American Academy of Allergy, Asthma, and Immunology. Doing this is helpful for everyone, he adds, but for those with a tendency toward sinus infections, it's particularly recommended.

To wash out your nasal passages, stand by the bathroom sink first thing in the morning, wash your hands with soap and water, then fill a bowl with 2 cups of water that feels as though it's around body temperature. Mix in ½ teaspoon salt and stir to dissolve. (If you are sensitive to iodine, use non-iodized salt.) Then pick up a small bulb syringe (available from your local drugstore) and squeeze out all the air. Put the narrow end into the saltwater solution and release the bulb to suck up the saltwater into the bulb. Squirt the water into the sink.

Now bend over the sink, squeeze the air out of the bulb once again, put the narrow end into the saltwater, release the bulb, and suck up the saltwater. Insert the tip of the syringe into one nostril—no farther than the width of your fingertip—and tilt the syringe tip toward the outer corner of your eye. Gently release the bulb and allow the water to gently squirt into your nose as you continue to lean over the sink.

Let the water drain out of your nostril back into the sink. Don't be alarmed if it comes out of your other nostril or your mouth. Both nostrils and the back of your mouth are all connected.

Repeat the procedure, switch nostrils, and then wash the second nostril twice. Wash out the bulb with fresh clean water several times, then store it, tip down, in a cup.

SQUIRT. "Nasal saline sprays can be very helpful," says Dr. Anderson. Use them throughout the day and particularly at night before bed. Avoid daily use of nasal vasoconstricting nose sprays, such as Afrin. If you use them for more than three days, you will become addicted. The nasal passages will swell and obstruct airway passages until the effect wears off—another three days.

FORGET OTC DECONGESTANTS. Over-the-counter decongestants can cause insomnia, says Dr. Anderson. If sleep is your objective, forget about taking 'em.

PRETREAT. Since your immune system responds to the allergen with inflammation and that's what swells shut your nasal passages, prevent the inflammation by using a prescription anti-inflammatory nasal spray, says Dr. Anderson. Brands inlclude Flonase, Nasonex, Veramyst, and Nasacort. All are effective.

LOOK FOR THE NEWER ANTIHISTAMINES. Older antihistamines can cause dry mouth or, when sold combined with decongestants, prevent sleep. "Newer antihistamines—including loratadine (generic Claritin), fexofenadine (generic Allegra), prescription Zyrtec, and prescription Clarinex don't interfere with sleep like some of the older ones do," says Dr. Anderson. Check with your doctor to see if one of them is right for you.

SHOWER WITH EUCALYPTUS. Head into the bathroom, turn on the shower, and fill the room with steam. Then sprinkle a half-dozen drops of essential oil of eucalyptus on your wet bath mitt, lather the mitt with an unscented soap, and wash your entire body from top to bottom. By the time you hit your feet, your nose will be breathing freely, your sinuses will be clear, and your throat will feel soothed and moisturized.

For an extra treat after you shampoo, use a few drops of eucalyptus in the final rinse for your hair. Keep it out of your eyes.

RINSE OFF. To keep pollen out of the bedroom, shower right before bed, use a dryer-dried towel, and don dryer-dried bedclothes.

HIDE OUT. Hot, dry, and windy weather can each send dust, pollen, and molds skittering through your windows at home, work, in your car—virtually everywhere. So stay indoors with windows closed when those conditions are present during your allergy season. Schedule shopping and outdoor activities when it's windless, cloudy, or even rainy. There's less pollen in the air.

CHECK THE POLLEN COUNT. If you have a pollen allergy, go to www.aaaai.org, click on "patients and consumers," then click on "pollen count" and follow the prompts to see what's pollinating in your area and how heavy the levels are. Plan outdoor activities when the counts are low; schedule indoor activities when the counts are high.

CLOSE WINDOWS IN THE EARLY MORNING. Pollen is usually emitted between 5:00 and 10:00 A.M. To avoid giving yourself a big dose before you even open your peepers, close windows the night before.

EXERCISE AFTER 10:00 A.M. You'll breathe better and get a better workout if you exercise after that 5:00 to 10:00 A.M. blast of pollen.

SCHEDULE VACATIONS DURING YOUR ALLERGY SEASON. Why not skip your allergy season altogether? Try vacationing in another part of the world while your allergens are blooming at home.

HIRE A LAWN PERSON. Mowing the grass stirs up a textbook's worth of pollens and molds, and raking leaves does the same thing. Hire a professional to do both—and suggest they wear a mask.

SCALD THE WASH AND RINSE WELL. A study at Yonsei University in South Korea looked at what it took to clean dust mites, dog dander, and tree pollen—three of the most common allergens—off your sheets.
 For dust mites it turns out that cold water killed 5 to 8 percent. Warm water killed 7 to 11 percent. Hot water—60°C or 140°F—killed 100 percent.
 For dog dander the results were similar—although nearly all allergens were removed at all wash temperatures when rinsing twice or more.
 For tree pollen using hot water was more effective than other temperatures. Rinsing at least once removed tree pollen at all temperatures.

WASH AND WASH AGAIN. Wash clothes and bedding weekly, says Dr. Anderson. It's the only way to stay on top of the allergens that disrupt sleep.

USE THE DRYER. Hanging laundry on the line allows a zillion pollens and molds to collect on sheets, clothes, and towels. When you fold your laundry, drop it into the laundry basket, and haul it back into your home, you're contaminating your house with millions upon millions of the very things to which you may be allergic.

REDUCE THE LOAD. To help reduce dust mites—which are everywhere in every home and aggravate every allergy—vacuum rugs and blinds often, says Dr. Anderson. Use a high-quality vacuum cleaner with a HEPA filter. Good vacuums will also pick up pet dander.

DOUBLE BAG. You're more likely to make a clean sweep of dust mites if you double bag your vacuum cleaner.

REDUCE HUMIDITY. Dust mites love moist areas. To discourage them from colonizing your home, use a dehumidifier to keep humidity below 50 percent, suggests Dr. Anderson. And don't forget to run an exhaust fan in the bathroom when you shower and in the kitchen when you cook.

INSTALL AIR-CONDITIONING. If you can afford it, it will help keep pollen out of your home and keep the humidity low to discourage dust mites. If you can't afford to air-condition your whole space, try using a room-size window air conditioner in your bedroom. It may help you sleep. Budget not up to even that? Then buy a HEPA filter and shape it to fit over your bedroom window screen, says Dr. Anderson. The pollens won't get in.

CHANGE FILTERS. On both cooling and heating systems. Those filters help trap allergens, but they'll get clogged unless they're changed every three months. HEPA filters are a bit pricey but are clearly the most effective.

BAN PETS. Not from your life, of course, but from your bedroom. A lot of people are apparently allergic to dog and cat dander without even being aware of it, says Dr. Anderson. They think their itchy nose and sneezing are due to something else altogether. But play it on the safe side. Let Beans or Spike or Rufus sleep in his own bed several rooms away from yours.

COVER THE MATTRESS. And especially the pillows. The cost of "allergy-proof" mattress and pillow covers can give you a heart attack, but those babies are worth their weight in gold. Dust mites are everywhere in everyone's home—and one of their preferential living spaces is your mattress. Zipping up the mattress and pillows in a mite-proof cover assures that the little critters can't interfere with your sleep.

BUY LEATHER. Leather does not collect dust mites the way fabric-covered furniture does, says Dr. Anderson. So buy leather-covered furniture where you can—vinyl where you can't.

LEAVE YOUR FLOORS BARE. Wall-to-wall carpeting harbors dust mites and pollen, while hardwood, tile, and vinyl don't. If you still crave something colorful on your floor, buy a few washable throw rugs and wash them weekly on a hot-water cycle.

KEEP AIR FRESH. In a study at the University of Washington in Seattle, researchers found that nearly half of all study participants with seasonal allergies also had allergy-type reactions to common household pollutants, such as household cleaning products, cigarette smoke, perfume, and aftershave. Why those with allergies were more likely to be sensitive to indoor pollutants isn't known.

MONITOR BATHROOM, KITCHEN, AND BASEMENT. These are three areas that tend to be more humid than the rest of the home. As a result, they're more prone to developing an allergy-triggering mold that will send spores winging their way through the entire house.

To eliminate mold, use a cleaning solution containing 5 percent bleach and a small amount of detergent. Moldy wallpaper or carpeting should be ditched.

Cancer

Sleep does not always come easily to 42-year-old Julie Silver. As the mother of three children, ages 7, 11, and 15, it seems as though someone's always awake and in need of attention. Someone's having nightmares; someone's worried about school; someone has to go to the bathroom.

"Sometimes it's Grand Central Station in here," she says, gesturing to her bedroom. "But what am I going to do? Say, 'No, you can't go to the bathroom?' "

She chuckles. "I'm a mom. This is what I *do*."

Taking care of her girls certainly is what she does. But as a doctor, an assistant professor at Harvard Medical School, and a breast cancer survivor, there are a few other things that Julie Silver, M.D., does, too.

For one thing, she understands that sleep isn't just beneficial for someone with cancer—it's inexorably intertwined with their healing. We now know, for example, that a lack of sleep seems to affect the activity of at least five different immune-system fighters, including natural killer cells, which are specialized cells specifically designed by your body to fight cancer.

Reel Therapy

To fill her mind with positive sleep-inducing images before bed, cancer survivor Julie Silver, M.D., likes to pop one of these films into her DVD player:

- *Meet the Parents*
- *You've Got Mail*
- *The River House*
- *50 First Dates*
- *Grease*
- *My Big Fat Greek Wedding*
- *Chocolat*
- *Father of the Bride*
- *The Wedding Planner*
- *Serendipity*

One Woman's Story

Pulling off her cycling jersey at her girlfriend's house after a 25-mile training ride for the 190-mile Pan-Mass Challenge across Massachusetts, 42-year-old Carolyn M. Kaelin, M.D., director of Harvard's Comprehensive Breast Health Center at Brigham and Women's Hospital, looked into a nearby mirror and noticed a tiny area of skin pulling inward on her right breast.

Moving back and forth so her image shifted around a warp in the mirror, Carolyn took a closer look at the area. There was no lump, and her skilled hands didn't feel anything out of the ordinary.

But, as a breast cancer surgeon, Carolyn had seen enough women with breast cancer to suspect that she had a problem. The next morning, after performing her first surgery of the day, she had a mammogram. It was normal. After performing her second surgery, she had an ultrasound. It seemed normal, but there was one little shape that didn't look quite right. She finished the remaining four surgeries on her schedule, then had a colleague remove a sample of her breast tissue for biopsy.

The next day, her colleague showed her the resulting slides and told her she had breast cancer. "It blindsided me," Carolyn says without hesitation. "I was young, I was healthy, I ate well, I exercised, I always tried to get a good night's sleep, and I didn't have anything compelling in my history.

"I think it does that to everybody. From an intellectual perspective, I pretty much knew I had breast cancer when I saw the skin retraction. So it wasn't a surprise when the chief of breast pathology came and told me. But..." She hesitates. "It was still a surprise. And to tell me I have the condition [for which] I've been treating people for so many years..." she says ruefully. "The irony did not escape me."

Once diagnosed, Carolyn moved swiftly. She had a lumpectomy. Then another. And another. Then, finally, a mastectomy.

"Breast-conserving surgery is, in an appropriate woman, a perfectly safe choice surgically," Carolyn says. "A mastectomy is not required for everyone. But my doctors came to find that I had three invasive breast cancers and a significant amount of adenocarcinoma. So I finally had a mastectomy."

By the time her surgical treatment was finished, Carolyn had had three lumpectomies, a mastectomy, and four other surgeries related to expanding chest tissue and inserting implants. All told, she had eight surgeries.

How did she sleep? Between discomfort from surgical treatment and stress related to diagnosis, treatment, her surgical workload, and the sheer immensity of her work on behalf of women everywhere, it's a miracle that Carolyn slept at all. But she did, and she slept well.

"I believe that when you're experiencing post-surgical pain, that is an appropriate time to take a physician-prescribed narcotic medication," says Carolyn. "I did as directed, and I slept."

Today, almost five years later, Carolyn is still on follow-up hormone therapy. She's developed an exercise rehab program, runs two-day intensive training sessions for trainers, and has written two books—including the acclaimed *Living through Breast Cancer*. She also spends a large part of her time in breast cancer survivor education outreach. Wherever she can lend a hand, she does—including helping to raise nearly $33 million dollars for cancer research from this year's Pan-Mass Challenge.

And she still sleeps well. But instead of help from narcotics, now her sleep is aided by exercise. "A good workout helps me get a good night's sleep," says the physician. "I'll walk the two miles to work, or, if I don't have a meeting, I'll run both ways. I also work in the gym with a trainer, and my husband, our two kids, and I walk to do all our grocery shopping."

Walk? With *groceries?*

"Five blocks each way," she says with a laugh, "and we live in a third-floor walkup."

"I need eight or nine hours of sleep at night now to function at the top of my game," she adds. "And I make sure I get it."

We also know that a lack of sleep is associated with a reduction in the level of melatonin, which is a natural antioxidant produced in your brain that is able to slow—or stop—the growth of tumors. Since melatonin reaches peak production levels at night while you sleep, tossing and turning half the night doesn't just leave you groggy in the morning, it may seriously affect your ability to fight cancer.

Who's Up?
50 percent of the 678,000 women who will develop cancer this year

Unfortunately, few of us will get a good night's sleep as we work through the suspicion that something is wrong and then deal with the testing, diagnosis, treatment, and recovery, says Dr. Silver. Fear, stress, pain, sadness, worry, disruption of the body's circadian rhythm, and the side effects of medication and treatment will see to that.

What can we do?

A lot. As Julie Silver writes in her book *After Cancer Treatment,* we can start with a walk, a prayer, a deep breath—and a commitment to nurture ourselves.

Sleep to Heal

While you sleep, your immune system produces some of your body's most effective cancer-fighting weapons. Here's how to make sure you get the sleep you need to maximize their production.

ACCEPT THE NEW NORMAL. "There's no five-year cure," says breast cancer survivor Julie Silver, M.D., an assistant professor at Harvard Medical School and author of *After Cancer Treatment*. "Even once you've been treated, you won't ever feel safe again. But you can learn to live with it."

When the fear wakes you up at night, counter it with positive images. Read books that keep your attention without having a plot that is too heavy. "I kept books by my bed that were very positive," says Dr. Silver, explaining that when you read, your brain literally takes a right turn away from what you've been thinking about, retools, and goes in a new direction. "So I really focused on putting positive images in my brain."

TRUST YOUR INSTINCTS. "You know your body best," says Dr. Silver. "No doctor will ever know it as well. Whether you think it's women's intuition or whatever, there's something that tells us when something's wrong. So when you think something's wrong, write down your symptoms and tell your doctor. And don't let anyone label you a hypochondriac. Trust your instincts."

MOVE. "Exercise improves sleep as effectively as benzodiazepines in some studies," reports Kalyanakrishnan Ramakrishnan, M.D., an associate professor at the University of Oklahoma Health Sciences Center. That makes exercise the number one treatment for insomnia in cancer survivors. But what also makes exercise the perfect prescription is the fact that it reduces the enormously debilitating fatigue that cancer survivors say is their chief complaint—and it cuts the eye-popping nighttime worry about recurrence.

In a Harvard Medical School study of more than 3,000 women with breast cancer, researchers found that those who walked 3 to 9 hours a week at a moderate (2 to 2.9 m.p.h.) pace reduced their risk of recurrence and death by 20 percent. If they walked 9 to 15 hours a week, they cut their risk by 50 percent. If they walked 15 to 24 hours a week, they cut their risk by a whopping 60 percent. More exercise than that, or more intense exercise, had no added benefit.

MEDICATE. "Pain is something that cancer patients really worry about," says Dr. Silver. Pain from tumors, pain from treatment, pain from the physical deconditioning that can take place through treatment, pain during recovery. Unfortunately, she adds, "the worry that pain is coming back can keep you awake as much as the pain does itself."

The trick is to stay on top of pain with regular doses of medication 24 hours a day. Women wake up in the morning and they feel good, so sometimes they don't take the pain medication their doctor has prescribed, or they don't take as much as they could, says Dr. Silver. They figure they can handle the little bit of pain they've got and save the medication for the big stuff. The problem is that the little stuff builds up during the day so that at night it's too big for the medication to handle. So take as much as your doctor prescribes, as often as she prescribes it.

GIVE UP NAPS. Since cancer and its treatment generally increase fatigue, chances are you'll start taking naps while you're undergoing treatment. But don't forget to give them up once you finish treatment. Otherwise, they'll begin to interfere with your ability to sleep at night.

ALERT YOUR DOCTOR. Sometimes your sleep is disrupted by the side effects of medication. So don't just dismiss insomnia as a natural consequence of middle-of-the-night worry over your health. Tell your doctor about it and ask what she thinks is the cause. Between the two of you, and maybe a night in a sleep lab, you may be able to get it fixed. If your chemotherapy is causing hot flushes, for example, a simple device like a Chillow—an ice-cooled pillow—and lowering your bedroom temperature may be enough to help you sleep through the night.

MAKE A SPECIFIC APPOINTMENT. Insomnia and fatigue are so common among cancer survivors that doctors sometimes don't pay attention when patients mention them. There's a lot going on during your appointment, and your doctor may tend to focus on other problems.

The way to get your doctor to focus on your sleep problem is to keep a sleep log (see page 104), says Dr. Silver. "Write down what's happening—what time you go to bed, how long it takes you to fall asleep, how often and when you wake up during the night, whether or not you fall back asleep, and what time you do," says Dr. Silver.

Then make a specific appointment that is devoted only to the sleep problem. That alone will impress your doctor of the seriousness of your sleep's disruption. But you should also pay attention to how you present the problem, she adds. "If a patient comes in and says, 'I'm really concerned about my sleep' rather than just saying, 'I haven't been sleeping,' that will trigger your doctor's concern."

PLAY BY THE RULES. The tenets of sleep medicine are well established, says Dr. Silver. And you can maximize your chances of a good night's sleep by sticking to them. Aim for between seven and eight hours of sleep a night. Avoid alcohol, exercise, and caffeine after 4:00 P.M. Shut down the computer early. Take a hot bath—not a shower—about an hour before bed to help you unwind. A light snack can help. Go to bed only when you're tired. If you wake up, lie in bed for only 20 to 30 minutes. After that, you should get up, go to another room, and return to bed only when you're sleepy again. Use your bedroom only for sleep or sex. Oh, all right—*and* for reading romance novels.

SHRUG IT OFF. When you find yourself wide awake at 3:00 A.M., just shrug it off. Okay, so you'll lose one night's sleep. Big deal. You have got enough to worry about.

FIGHT NIGHTTIME NAUSEA. Grate one tablespoon of gingerroot into a cup of hot water. Steep for 10 minutes, then sip. Forget the packaged stuff—you can't count on the same amount of active ingredient in each and every tea bag.

USE THE 4-STEP METHOD. A study at Harvard Medical School found that women who experienced tamoxifen-induced hot flushes had significantly fewer hot flushes during cancer treatment when they practiced the relaxation response pioneered by Herbert Benson, M.D., a cardiologist who heads the Mind/Body Medical Institute in Boston.

In general, the response involves these four steps:

1. Choose a word that has deep personal meaning for you, such as "peace."

2. Close your eyes and focus your attention on the word. Repeat it silently to yourself. When your attention wanders, as it will, gently bring it back to the word.

3. Take a deep breath and exhale. Begin to consciously relax each of your muscles from your face to your toes.

4. When you're finished, continue to focus on your chosen word for another 10 to 15 minutes.

Then allow yourself to gently move into sleep.

TREAT WHAT YOU CAN TREAT. Sometimes you have an underlying condition—arthritis, back pain, or snoring, for example—that has always troubled your sleep but was never a big deal. Then all of a sudden you add chemotherapy to the mix and find that sleep is a thing of the past. There's not a lot you can do about the chemotherapy, but you can do something about the arthritis, back pain, or snoring. Tell your oncologist about the underlying problem and ask him what treatment will work best with your chemotherapy. Chances are, just treating the underlying problem will reduce what's disturbing you enough to let you sleep.

DITCH NEWS AND STUPID OPINIONS. Negative words and images are not going to help you sleep. So—at least in the hours before bed—avoid TV news programs and the amazing collection of opinionated talk-show hosts who make their living stirring up anger and controversy. Allow yourself to get ready for bed without their voices in your head.

STRIKE A BALANCE. Women aren't used to nurturing themselves or putting themselves first. But sleep is so necessary for healing that you have to do it. If the dog's snoring wakes you up, put him in another room. If your partner's snoring wakes you, whether it's just a seasonal allergy, a cold, or even sleep apnea, help him get treatment. If he refuses to cooperate, put him in another room, too.

"One thing that really kept me up, and keeps me up today, is my kids," admits Dr. Silver. "My daughter has been in three times this week with nightmares. She's seven years old and it's September, and she's just starting school again. So she has a lot of things going on in her mind. But she wakes me up, and it's hard to go back to sleep.

The thing is, you can't just turn off being a mom. Yes, you need to nurture yourself so you'll heal. But your children are going through cancer, too. They're worried about you, about themselves, about how everything has changed. So you need to nurture yourself, but within the constraints of reality.

"You can't just send your kid back to bed with her fear," says Dr. Silver, "but I would use every trick to reassure my kids so that I could get them to sleep." She'd also use some parenting tactics that, under normal circumstances, would horrify her—like promising to buy them gifts if they would go to sleep.

"Desperate times call for desperate measures," says Dr. Silver. "And when you're having cancer treatment and you're desperately trying to heal, well, maybe that isn't exactly the way you would parent under normal circumstances. But you do what you need to do to get them"—and you—"to sleep."

CONNECT. Reach out to friends and family. Call your best friend, sit with a neighbor in your backyard as she cuts back your roses, ask your mom to come make you lunch, have friends from your spiritual community drop by. Feel a part of that rich network of human sustenance.

ASK FOR PRAYER. "I asked people to pray for me at 9:00 P.M. every night," says Dr. Silver. "That was after I'd put my kids to bed and I was alone in my room, usually in pain, trying to sleep.

"I was incredibly lonely and incredibly scared. My usual routine had been changed. I went to bed much earlier, and when I went to bed, I was very worried and very lonely."

She hesitates. "You know, cancer's a very lonely disease. I have a wonderful, wonderful husband, awesome kids, a great family, terrific friends. But cancer's a lonely disease, and you fight it by yourself.

"To feel surrounded and uplifted by prayer—it helps."

Pain

Yes, 1 out of every 10 of us have spent at least one day in pain during the last month—and 86 percent of us didn't sleep because of it. Low back pain is the most common cause—frequently joined by migraine headaches, joint pain, aching, or stiffness.

"Pain is a nearly constant companion throughout our lives," says Julie K. Silver, M.D., an assistant professor of physical medicine and rehabilitation at Harvard Medical School and author of *Super Healing*. And in certain conditions like migraines and fibromyalgia, it looks as though women are more susceptible to pain than men. No one knows precisely why, she adds, "but it likely has a biological basis that we don't fully understand."

The differences between how men and women experience pain is

One Woman's Story

JANE ROBERTS: Sleepless in L.A.

Waiting tables at a hip Italian nightspot in Los Angeles was tough for 42-year-old Jane Roberts. For six to eight hours a night, she'd heft a heavy tray loaded with plates and bowls full of food, plus assorted beverages, and head out from the kitchen to one of two interior dining rooms, three bars, or a huge outdoor patio that sat over 300 people.

"I literally ran around for hours," sighs Jane. "I walked at least five miles a night, but I wouldn't feel the pain until I got home and sat down. Then I'd just think, 'Wow. My body really hurts.' "

The aches and pains made sleeping difficult. But an over-the-counter sleep aid and a long hot bath before bed helped relax her tortured muscles. And for those exquisitely nasty spots that still seemed to think she was in the midst of balancing trays—a topical pain reliever rubbed into her skin.

The Vitamin D Effect

A new study at the Mayo Clinic reveals that a quarter of those who experienced chronic pain had low levels of vitamin D—and that those who did needed nearly twice the narcotics to control their pain than those with adequate vitamin D. They also needed medication nearly twice as long.

If you have chronic pain, ask your doctor for a blood test to check your levels of vitamin D. If they're low, she can recommend a prescription supplement that, taken once or twice a week for four to six weeks, will resolve the problem—and possibly some of your pain.

intriguing. A review of pain studies by researchers at the University of Tulsa suggests that it's possible that women's neurochemistry sets them up to be more sensitive, and a review of imaging studies of the brain at the famed Karolinska Institute in Stockholm demonstrates that both women and men have a clear biological difference in how their biochemistry responds to pain.

Still other studies reveal that a woman's pain threshold and pain tolerance varies with the stage of her menstrual cycle. Even more intriguing, a review of laboratory studies found that males—at least male rodents—not only have a lower sensitivity to pain, they also have a built-in painkilling system that generates far more natural painkillers than that of their female counterparts.

The result? Men experience pain less intensely—which may explain why studies show that women report pain twice as often as men.

> "I go in my mind into our summer house or another house I know and try to remember everything I see as I walk through it. I do that a lot."
>
> —SUSAN JONES

Now, a number of scientists will quibble about the relationship between rats and men and tell you that the notion that rats and men have interchangeable parts isn't necessarily scientifically accurate.

But if some know-it-all brother, husband, son, or significant other suggests that you're a wimp about pain, our position is that you should feel free to announce that women are biologically built to withstand a lot more pain than any man is ever likely to see.

Whether it aches, stings, shoots, burns, stabs, tingles, or practically knocks you unconscious, few of us can sleep through pain.

What Should I Do?

Most pain, particularly the kind that wakes us in the night, is related to muscles and joints—muscle strains, tendonitis, osteoarthritis, that kind of thing. It hurts, but it's not usually life threatening. So the rule of thumb is to handle it yourself and wait two weeks to see if it disappears. If it doesn't, call your doctor.

Other types of pain require more immediate attention, says Julie K. Silver, M.D. Here's what they are:

- Pain after some kind of accident, such as a fall, should be immediately checked by a doctor even if there are no outward signs that something is wrong. If your doctor is not immediately available, head for the emergency room or call 911.

- Pain that is new or severe and occurs in your head, chest, or abdomen should immediately be checked by your doctor. Call immediately, and make sure whoever relays your message to the doctor understands that you're not talking about a stubbed toe.

- Pain accompanied by numbness, weakness, or dizziness should be checked as soon as possible. Call your doctor's office for an appointment, and make sure you get one within a day or two.

Three Ways to Hurt

Pain is the immediate response by your body to get your attention and crank up the body's protective machinery. That machinery will either get you moving—away from something that has hurt you, for example—or it will initiate an internal cascade of chemical messages that will get something fixed that you may not even be aware needs fixing.

But that pertains to what's called once-and-done pain. Once whatever started it is taken care of, it disappears.

Chronic pain is a whole other ball game. When pain is chronic, it's triggered either by direct nerve activation—for example, when the inflammation of arthritis sets off an insidious ache—by damaged or injured nerves firing off pain messages because they no longer know how to do their job, or by changes in a section of your brain that has learned to take nonpain messages and upgrade them so that other parts of your brain read them as pain.

The result? Pain when there isn't a cause, or when the cause has actually disappeared.

Unfortunately, chronic pain affects 1 in 3 of us—and 90 percent of those who have it can't sleep.

Overcoming Nighttime Pain

Pain not only interferes with your ability to get a good night's sleep, it actually disrupts the sleep you *do* get by encouraging your brain to wake you up throughout the night. That's because pain and sleep share common biological pathways, says Julie K. Silver, M.D., an assistant professor of physical medicine and rehabilitation at Harvard Medical School. So even if your eyes remain shut most of the night, chances are your brain still isn't getting the deep, restorative sleep it needs. As a result, you wake up in the morning feeling far from refreshed. Also, sleep deprivation actually increases your sensitivity to the pain. Yeah, you read that right. So pain = less sleep = more pain.

Want to escape from that nasty little loop and get some sleep? Here's what Dr. Silver prescribes.

LISTEN TO YOUR BODY. When pain first raises the alarm that something's wrong, pay attention. Precisely where is the pain? On a scale of 0 to 10, with 0 being no pain and 10 indicating the worst possible pain imaginable, where is your pain? What makes your pain worse? Do any other symptoms accompany it?

TRACK YOUR PAIN. If the pain's not severe—and remember, severe pain requires a doctor's immediate intervention—keep a pain log and track the pain for a month, says Dr. Silver. Jot down when it occurs, its rank on a scale of 1 to 10, and what makes it better or worse.

MEDICATE. Whether it's delivered as a pill, patch, cream, or injection, medication can be God's gift to the hurting. Ranging from acetaminophen and lidocaine patches to low-dose antidepressants and muscle relaxants, the arsenal is awesome. But every one has side effects, and not every one works in every situation. Work with your doctor to find the best approach.

ENLIST YOUR DOCTOR'S HELP. There is no virtue in bearing pain. Its your body's alarm system that something is wrong. So get to the person who can help you figure out what your body's trying to say: your doctor.

DON'T DO ANYTHING STUPID. While you're waiting to see your doctor, don't aggravate your pain. If you have hip pain every time you run, don't run. Walk instead.

HEAT IT UP. Try applying a hot pack to the area in which the pain occurs for 20 minutes a day.

COOL IT DOWN. Try a cold pack for 20 minutes once a day. Wrap the area in a towel to make sure the outside of the pack doesn't touch your skin. Cold packs reduce inflammation and provide a temporary numbing effect.

HAVE A MASSAGE. Schedule one session a week and see how you feel.

OR TRY ACUPUNCTURE. Just keep in mind that it takes six to eight sessions before you'll notice any effect. This is not a quick fix.

MOVE. Have your doctor refer you to a physical therapist who can design a personal movement program that targets the area in pain. Also, work with your therapist to get an aerobic exercise program that works for you.

STAY ON TOP. Treat pain aggressively early in the day, says Dr. Silver, and you'll be more likely to control it more effectively and with less medication throughout the day and evening. Play tough girl and let it remain at a low ebb all day and it's sure to build. Then, when everything's quiet and you're lying in bed trying to sleep, it'll get you but good.

PRAY. A survey by researchers at Stanford University Medical Center found that 62 percent of women under 50 who had pain prayed for relief. Seventy-one percent of women over 50 prayed. The result? Prayer worked in half of those who tried it. Amazingly, it relieved pain just as well as prescription meds.

SEE THE PAIN DOCTOR. If you still can't get on top of your pain, schedule an appointment with a doctor who specializes in treating pain.

Coping
with Loss

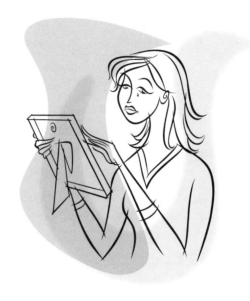

When Debbie's husband, John, died of pancreatic cancer at age 48, she and her two children were left with a sense of things unsaid. Death had come more quickly than any of them had expected, and for months afterward Debbie searched through John's papers, pockets, and drawers hoping for some note that said good-bye.

Sadly, more than half of us will lose our partners **by age 65.**

There was nothing.

Grief is hard. There is no easy way to move through it. Most of us who lose someone we love will feel bruised right down to our soul. We'll feel worry, fear, sadness, guilt, anger, frustration, confusion, and loneliness. Some psychologists say that those feelings are stages through which we move. But the truth is, moving through those stages is circular. We'll begin to move on, spot a glove or a book left behind, and slip right back into a puddle of despair.

A Time of Turbulent Emotions

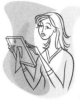 Unfortunately, a consequence of these uncontrollable feelings is something that makes it even harder to handle: Most of us simply don't sleep. We lie down, turn out the light, close our eyes—and our minds remain sharply alert. And when we finally slip into unconsciousness, we frequently wake through the night.

Disrupted sleep makes it harder to handle our grief, our lives, and even the day-to-day duties of making the bed or paying the bills. And it may also affect our health. In a study of 4,395 married couples at the University of Glasgow, for example, when one spouse died, the risk of the other spouse dying from anything ranging from heart disease, stroke, and cancer to accidents and violence increased by 27 percent.

SUCKER-PUNCHED

Grief is most likely to be intense when something—a memory, a smell, a glimpse of mutual friends—unexpectedly catches you off guard.

"The anniversary dates and holidays that are anticipated and dreaded are very often not as bad as you might expect," says Belleruth Naparstek, M.S., a therapist who lost her husband a couple of years ago. "But the first time you go to the cleaners and find your dead husband's beautifully pressed shirts on hangers under the transparent plastic bag—that will take the breath out of you."

When it happens, you're guaranteed to toss and turn. But Naparstek suggests you don't even try to avoid these lightning bolts of pain. "It's better to feel the grief, breathe through it, and know this is what happens," she says, explaining that it's the only way to keep moving forward.

DO YOU NEED HELP?

For the past several years an unfortunate claim from a psychology student's paper has been floating around newspapers, magazines, and even some professional journals. It concludes that grief counseling or therapy with a trained therapist prolongs the grieving process and harms rather than helps.

What harms rather than helps is the misinformation. The truth, as acknowledged in reputable medical journals, is that grief counseling *does* help the bereaved move through the grieving process. And it's particularly helpful for the 15 percent of us who, for whatever reason, have gotten stuck in our grief and are unable to move on.

The warning signs that grieving has gone beyond normal bounds and signals you're in need of a helping hand include:

- A sense of emptiness

- Feeling that part of you died along with the deceased

- "Excessive" yearning for the deceased

- An absence of grief

- Delayed grief

- Conflicted grief

- Chronic grief

- Avoiding reminders of the deceased

- Continually thinking or dreaming of the deceased

- Using alcohol or drugs to avoid painful feelings

- Suicidal thoughts

If you experience any of these symptoms, ask your doctor to recommend a local psychologist who is trained to offer grief therapy.

The Biochemistry of Grief

Researchers are still trying to figure out the exact relationship between grief, sleep, and mortality. Right now all they really know is that grief seems to suppress the immune system and that there's a huge rise in adrenaline in response to the death of someone you love.

"Adrenaline is the biochemical that causes sleep loss," explains Cleveland therapist Belleruth Naparstek, M.S., who lost her husband, Art, a couple of years ago. "It's triggered by intense loss, and in the case of a deceased spouse, also from survivor terror."

Survivor terror comes from the sudden realization that you are left with all the things your spouse used to do, she explains. Whatever it was—banking, cooking, investing, shopping—you're the one who has to pick up the load and carry it. In most cases you'll do fine. In others you'll have a learning curve. And whether the responsibilities are doable or not, you'll have to figure out how you're going to get the time to integrate them into your already existing stack of responsibilities.

HOW CAN FRIENDS HELP?

Let your friends take some of the responsibility from your shoulders. You will sleep easier just knowing they're willing to do whatever you need. Here's some of what you can ask them to do:

- Listen.

- Don't tell you things will get better.

- Write thank you notes.

- Answer the phone.

- Tell you things will get better.

- Share stories about your partner, especially funny ones.

- Shuttle you around to banks, lawyers, and the funeral home.

- Walk the dog.

- Just sit beside you.

A COMPANION FOR THE JOURNEY

Sometimes you don't feel ready to hang out with friends or join a support group. If that's the case, open one of these books and allow the authors—all widows—to share their journey through grief.

- *I Wasn't Ready to Say Goodbye* by Brook Noel

- *Being a Widow* by Lynn Caine

- *Companion through the Darkness: Inner Dialogues on Grief* by Stephanie Ericsson

- *I'm Grieving As Fast As I Can* by Linda Feinberg

- *The Road Taken: A Memoir—One VW Bus, One Widow, Nine Kids* by Therese Powers Kramer

- *A Widow's Walk: A Memoir of 9/11* by Marian Fontana

That alone can keep anybody charged up and highly adrenalized well into the night.

"Grief can also trigger a lot of circular thinking," says Naparstek. The how-will-I-pay-the-mortgage thoughts. The how-will-I-raise-the-children thoughts. The what-should-I-have-done-differently thoughts.

"Even if there's no guilt involved," she says knowingly, "you're going to be thinking it."

Trying to figure out how you relate to others after a loss will also keep your adrenaline pumping, she adds. "It's not just that you've lost your place in the community as part of a couple, your own preferences change." One-on-one girlfriend talks about issues you might have with your spouse are no longer the norm for you.

"Whether people do it to you or you do it to yourself," she concludes, "there's a whole realignment of your social network."

The one thing that really kept Naparstek up, however, was all of the incredibly inappropriate or insensitive things people said. "Dealing with stupid people is huge," says Naparstek. "Especially within the first year, when you're feeling particularly skinless.

'*God doesn't give you anything more than you can handle*,' " she mimics. Or "*It's such a loss to the community*." Even, '*Look at what you have to be thankful for.*' People who don't even know you come up, wring their hands, look at you with pity, and make some insensitive remark," she says in exasperation. "You just want to *smack* them.

"One day I was in the gym reading the *New York Times* on the treadmill, and someone I knew only marginally came up to me and wanted me to 'share my feelings.' "

Why do they do it?

She sighs. "They're terrified it's going to happen to them, and they're projecting their own anxiety. Or they always wanted to be your best friend and this is their opportunity."

Either way, says the therapist, "you spend the energy fending them off, then stay up all night feeling like you've been assaulted."

10 Stupid Things People Say to New Widows

- *I know how you feel.*
- Think of all the good times.
- He'll be a great loss to the community.
- *I know how you feel.*
- Call me if you need anything.
- It was God's will.
- It's time to get on with your life.
- You'll feel better in a couple of weeks.
- My dog died last week, too.
- *I know how you feel.*

How to Sleep Alone

Nothing will ease your grief—at least, not for a while. But these tips will help you sleep, and sleep will help you heal.

JOURNAL. Limit writing to 15 minutes a day, and just write about how you feel. Periodically read back through what you've written. Over time you'll be able to see how you've moved through the grieving process. Somewhere around 80 percent of us will move through the worst of our grief within a year.

NURTURE YOURSELF. Pay attention to your body's needs. Prepare balanced meals, and serve them on your best china and linens. Exercise for 30 minutes every day, even if it's just a walk with the dog. And every morning center yourself in a prayer of gratitude for the people in your life, the sunshine outside your window, and the fact that you can make a difference in the lives of others.

CONSULT SOME EXPERTS. Check with your attorney and a financial consultant about the effects a death has on your legal and financial situation. No, you don't want to deal with it. On the other hand, you'll sleep better knowing exactly what will—or won't—be coming at you in the months ahead.

USE GUIDED IMAGERY. "Mind/body stuff really works in helping you get to sleep," says therapist Belleruth Naparstek, M.S. "The imagery has enough cognitive recruitment to seduce the brain into seeing and thinking about other things, while the voice tone, pacing, music, and images will persuade your parasympathetic nervous system that it's time to calm down. It will shut down the adrenaline and shoot some calming hormones into your nervous system."

Slip a CD of guided imagery into your CD player, snuggle into bed, turn out the lights, and follow the imagery into sleep.

BAN THE BOTTLE. Alcohol simply prolongs the grieving process and makes it harder to get good, restorative sleep.

SCHEDULE A MASSAGE. "Massage interrupts the neurohormones connected with sleeplessness and almost manually imposes sleep on you," says Naparstek. "If you can't afford a massage, go to a massage school. You can get one there for $15."

GET WHAT YOU NEED. "For some people six months of Ambien is a good thing," says Naparstek. "If you need to take medication to interrupt the adrenalization of your life, so be it."

FIND NEW FRIENDS. Preferably other widows. Several women who belonged to the same church in Spring Hill, Florida, banded together after the death of their husbands and called themselves the Merry Widows. One was an artist, another a real estate agent, and two others were homemakers.

At first they weren't merry at all—like everybody else, they were devastated by their losses. But gradually as they met for lunch or dinner, picked each other up for church, and brought takeout or chicken soup to those who were sick, things changed. They joked—with a sometimes macabre humor that could startle those still married folks who overheard them—providing an understanding and caring for one another that soothed their adrenalized state.

READ. Books on grieving, particularly memoirs of survivors, can reassure you that many of the intense feelings keeping you up will someday ease.

WRITE A LETTER. What would you tell your partner if you had a chance? Even if you don't share the letter with anyone, the process of writing it may help you unload some of that adrenaline. If you're angry, feel free to vent.

ACCEPT YOUR GRIEF. Allow yourself to move through all the emotions associated with grieving—sadness, longing, guilt, anger, betrayal, the whole range of passionate emotion that allows you to be the loving, caring person you are. Don't try to stiff-upper-lip it. You'll only make getting to sleep harder, prolonging the grieving process.

BE CLEAR. So many people will want to talk with you about your spouse and your grief. Friends will want to process their own grief by talking about it over and over. Be tough and tell them very clearly to leave you alone. Same goes for those whom who know only slightly. "I got very comfortable saying, `I don't want to talk about this,' " says Naparstek.

COLLECT THE STUPID THINGS PEOPLE SAY. Write them down, share them with close friends, and joke about them. "I had a friend—a nurse—whose husband died of a heart attack," Naparstek says. "I knew that she'd had a snootful of all the things people say. So I called and said, `Wanna get together for dinner? I'm buying. And we can talk about all the stupid things people say to new widows!' " She laughs. "We had a blast!"

Sleep Disorders

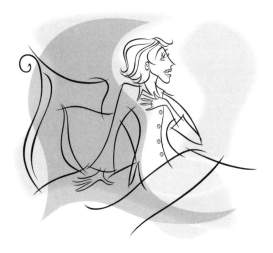

There are more than 80 sleep disorders that can prevent you from having a good night's sleep. Topping the list of conditions are narcolepsy, restless legs syndrome, and sleep apnea. And sleep is not the only area that suffers. How you function during the day is deeply affected as well. Some women with narcolepsy will avoid having an orgasm during sex because they're afraid it will trigger a temporary paralysis that sometimes accompanies the condition. And women with sleep apnea will wake so exhausted that morning sex seems like a dream from the distant past. Fortunately, there are ways to overcome these conditions—and rediscover the person you've always been.

> Sleep apnea affects **women** of **any age** and **weight, not just** the **overweight** middle-aged man.

Narcolepsy

When Gloria dozed off in the front pew of her Spring Hill, Florida, church for the fourth Sunday in a row, she was mortified.

"Was I snoring?" she anxiously asked a friend.

Reassured that she hadn't made anything more than a gentle snuffling sound, she relaxed. And promptly fell asleep.

Narcolepsy isn't the easiest sleep disorder to live with. It frequently begins when a woman is in her twenties but is usually misdiagnosed for an average of 15 years. Consequently, it is often mistakenly related to a condition that pops up during the perimenopausal years (see "Perimenopause: The 24/7 Woman," on page 109).

Narcolepsy is apparently caused by a genetic glitch that prevents the body from either absorbing or producing enough of the neurochemical hypocretin. In either case the brain's sleep/wake switch behaves erratically, and those with the condition unexpectedly fall asleep multiple times throughout the day and, conversely, wake up unexpectedly throughout the night.

"It's difficult to stay awake and difficult to stay asleep," says neurologist Eveline Honig, M.D., director of the Narcolepsy Network. "The quality of sleep is poor, so people are exhausted all the time. And that makes it twice as hard to function."

"Whenever I can't sleep, I use a technique a doctor once suggested. I breathe in slowly and hold it for the same amount of time that I take to inhale, and I do this continuously until I begin to feel relaxed. Focusing on my breathing clears my head so I can go back to sleep."

—CHRISTINE LAGANA

Complicating things is the fact that those with the condition can be unable to move when they wake, a kind of paralysis that can last from one second to 20 minutes.

Even more challenging are the hallucinations that some people experience as they emerge from sleep—the dog you've been dreaming about bites you, for example—especially since it's almost impossible for the person with narcolepsy to tell whether it was a hallucination or it really happened. Then there's the tendency among some to collapse into a temporary state of paralysis whenever they become excited. Because of this, some women with narcolepsy avoid having orgasms during sex.

"It's hard," says Dr. Honig. "Narcolepsy affects how you behave, how you work, and all your relationships. But the worst thing is when people see someone with narcolepsy fall asleep. They simply assume that they're lazy."

Do You Have Narcolepsy?

If you experience any of the following symptoms, check in with your primary-care physician.

- Are you falling asleep at inappropriate times and places?

- Do you have vivid dreams or hallucinations as you fall asleep or wake up?

- Are you ever unable to move or speak when falling asleep or waking up?

- Have you experienced sudden muscle weakness that may cause you to collapse?

Tinker with Your Brain

Although those with narcolepsy can't do a lot to change how others may view them, they can do a lot to manage their disorder. Here's how.

NAP. "Sometimes narcolepsy can be managed entirely by naps alone," says neurologist Eveline Honig, M.D., Director of the Narcolepsy Network. Although it may sound a bit odd to prescribe naps for someone who falls asleep all the time, sleep experts suggest you take two naps a day—one at lunchtime and one around 4:00 P.M. The naps should last no more than 15 to 30 minutes. That's enough to improve your alertness significantly, while longer naps can make you feel groggy.

STAY ON A REGULAR SCHEDULE. If you keep to a routine, it will help that little switch in your brain know whether it should be on or off.

CONSIDER MEDS. Stimulants like methylphenidate (Ritalin) and modafinil (Provigil) frequently help you stay alert.

WATCH WHAT GOES IN YOUR MOUTH. In general, carbs make you sleepy while protein makes you more alert, says Dr. Honig. The best thing to do is keep a food diary noting the food you eat, the time you eat it, what you were doing afterward, and whether you had any subsequent symptoms. Then simply avoid foods that you know make you sleepy.

AVOID ALCOHOL. It screws up everything. If your brain has trouble recognizing normal sleep/wake signals, alcohol is the wild card that will confuse it forever.

JOIN THE NARCOLEPSY NETWORK. Their Web site and newsletter offer links to the latest information, research, and other types of support around the country. They also sponsor a national "sleep in." Go to sleep.rd.com and click on "Narcolepsy."

Restless Legs

Restless legs syndrome is a condition that ranges from a creepy-crawly sensation that runs up and down your legs to quivers, jerks, pins and needles, numbness, pain, or a burning sensation. It affects millions of individuals every day, and their chief complaint is difficulty falling asleep—and staying asleep. That's because that is when these sensations typically occur. And unfortunately, many people who have RLS also have trouble controlling sudden limb movements, which can occur every 20 to 30 seconds all night long—a major sleep disrupter.

Twenty percent of pregnant women also suffer from RLS. If you're expecting, "delivery is the real remedy," says Grace Pien, M.D., a sleep researcher at the University of Pennsylvania's Center for Sleep and Respiratory Neurobiology.

DO YOU HAVE RESTLESS LEGS SYNDROME (RLS)?

RLS can be experienced in varying degrees, from mild to severe. Here's what to look for:

- When you sit or lie down, do you have a strong desire to move your legs?

- Does your desire to move your legs feel impossible to resist?

- Have you ever used the words unpleasant, creepy crawly, creeping, itching, pulling, or tugging to describe your symptoms to others?

- Does your desire to move often occur when you are resting or sitting still?

- Does moving your legs make you feel better?

- Do you complain of these symptoms more at night?

- Do you keep your bed partner awake with the jerking movements of your legs?

- Do you ever have involuntary leg movements while you are awake?

- Are you tired or unable to concentrate during the day?

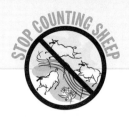

Kick the Restless Legs

Here's what will help.

WALK BEFORE BED. Don't do anything too aerobic, because that will keep you up. Just take a nice, quiet stroll around the block before you turn in.

STRETCH. Doing leg stretches for five minutes or so right before you hop into bed will help settle your legs.

WARM YOUR LEGS. Apply heat over your lower legs when you lie down. A microwavable heat pack stuffed with fragrant herbs is perfect. When it cools, you don't even have to get up. You can toss it under the bed, turn out the light, and head into dreamland.

AVOID ANTIHISTAMINES. Over-the-counter sleep aids that contain anti-histamines will make restless legs worse. Avoid them under any circumstances.

CHECK IRON AND FOLATE LEVELS. Even when you take vitamins, some women develop an anemia that will cause leg cramps and restless legs. Your doctor can run a simple blood test that will reveal inadequate levels. If levels are low, she may prescribe an iron or B-complex supplement.

BEEF UP YOUR DIET. During pregnancy, eat a diet rich in red meat, eggs, and whole grains to maintain adequate iron and folate levels.

STAY OUT OF SMOKY ROOMS. Studies show that pregnant women who are exposed to tobacco smoke have double the risk of restless legs.

Sleep Apnea

If you wake in the morning feeling sleepy, irritable, sad, forgetful, and headachy, there's a good chance that you have sleep apnea, a sleep-related breathing disorder that affects 20 million of us—particularly when we're pregnant.

When you have the disorder, your breathing actually stops or gets very shallow as you sleep. Hundreds of times every night, your breathing may pause for 10 or more seconds, depriving your body of oxygen and increasing your heart rate. You may awaken slightly as you struggle to take a breath. But the next morning, says Rochelle Goldberg, M.D., president of the American Sleep Apnea Association (ASAA), you may not recall any of your nighttime awakenings.

There are three types of sleep apnea: obstructive, central, and complex. Obstructive sleep apnea, or OSA, is the most common, accounting for approximately 90 percent of all sleep apnea. OSA occurs when the soft tissue in the back of your throat relaxes and blocks the passage of air until your airway opens—often with a loud choking or gasping sound—and you begin to breathe again.

Approximately 10 percent of people with apnea suffer from central sleep apnea, in which the brain "forgets" to signal the airway muscles to breathe. Many people with central sleep apnea have some other disease, such as congestive heart failure, brain disease, stroke, or hypothyroidism (low thyroid function), and researchers are still working to discover the reason for the association. In some cases, though, the underlying cause is unknown.

A third type, complex sleep apnea, is rare. It's a combination of obstructive and central sleep apnea. For people with complex sleep apnea, the brain not only fails to send a message to breathe, but the airways are obstructed as well.

Untreated sleep apnea has been linked to a number of health concerns, including hypertension, heart disease, stroke, diabetes, and weight gain. And since poor sleep results in slower reflexes, poor concentration, and the risk of nodding off behind the wheel, it also puts you at risk for driving accidents.

Unfortunately, however, many people just don't take the snoring of sleep apnea seriously, and 80 to 90 percent of us with sleep apnea are undiagnosed and untreated, according to the American Academy of Sleep Medicine.

"Sleep apnea is far less likely to be diagnosed in women than in men. That's a real challenge we have to overcome," says Dr. Goldberg.

There are many reasons why fewer women get evaluated and treated than men. Women may blame their daytime sleepiness on other causes, such as insomnia or chronic fatigue. Women also tend to be more embarrassed by their loud snoring, which can keep them from discussing their condition with their doctors. Also, men tend to sleep more soundly than women, so a woman's breathing pauses and loud snoring may not get noticed as readily by their male partners.

DO YOU HAVE SLEEP APNEA?

Here are the key signs to watch for:

- Do you snore loudly? About half of all people who snore loudly have obstructive sleep apnea (OSA). It's a sign that your airway is partially blocked.

- What's your neck size? The size of your neck can be a telltale sign. Women with OSA often have a neck size of more than 16 inches (17 inches for men).

- Are you waking often to take bathroom breaks? "Most adults who don't drink lots of water before bed and are not uncontrolled diabetics or on high doses of water pills should not have to wake repetitively to use the bathroom," says Rochelle Goldberg, M.D., president of the American Sleep Apnea Association.

Block That Snore

There are a variety of treatments available for sleep apnea, but what works for you will depend on the severity of your problem and your commitment to treatment. Making the following lifestyle changes will help you get a good night's sleep.

KEEP THAT AIRWAY TONED. Avoid alcohol, sedatives, sleeping pills, and any medication that relaxes the central nervous system, making it more difficult to keep your throat open while sleeping.

DUMP POUNDS. Work with your doctor on a weight-loss plan if you are overweight. Even a small drop in weight can improve your symptoms. Unfortunately, sleep apnea can make losing weight more difficult because it interferes with leptin and ghrelin, two brain chemicals that signal the body that it's full.

QUIT SMOKING. Add sleep apnea to the long list of reasons why you should kick the habit. If you have sleep apnea, your body is hungry for oxygen. Unfortunately, smoking will reduce the amount of oxygen available.

SLEEP ON YOUR SIDE. You're more likely to snore loudly when you sleep on your back. Try special pillows that make back sleeping impossible or at least uncomfortable. For example, you can wedge a pillow stuffed with tennis balls behind your back to make rolling over unpleasant.

SEE A SLEEP SPECIALIST. If your apnea is moderate to severe or you've made lifestyle changes and you still have symptoms of sleep apnea, then you need to see a sleep specialist who can observe and evaluate your sleep and help you find the best solution for you and your problem. A sleep doctor will check your mouth, nose, and throat and make a recording of what happens with your breathing while you sleep. This may require an overnight stay at a sleep center.

Often, sleep specialists recommend continuous positive airway pressure (CPAP), which is the most common treatment for sleep apnea. With CPAP you wear a face mask over your nose that blows pressurized air into your airway to keep it open while you sleep. However, this is not a long-term solution: Sleep apnea will return as soon as you stop relying on CPAP.

Many people avoid seeking professional help for sleep apnea because they know about CPAP and fear using it, says Rochelle Goldberg, M.D., president of the American Sleep Apnea Association. But the treatment works well and can be truly lifesaving for some people. Many patients discover that they finally achieve their best sleep in years once they start using the device.

To help those with loud snoring and mild to moderate sleep apnea, there is a mouthpiece that holds the jaw and tongue in a position that aids breathing. It's the second line of therapy for most patients. While it's not as successful as CPAP, the mouthpiece is an option for people who aren't comfortable using the breathing mask. It's also more portable, so people who travel frequently often prefer it to CPAP.

Surgery is also an option for some. The type of surgery will depend on the severity of the problem, as well as the underlying cause. Your sleep center may refer you to an ear, nose, and throat doctor for an evaluation.

Nightmares

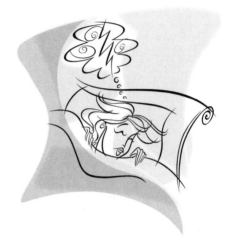

Cold blue chills run down your body. An electric charge snakes across your skin. Your pupils dilate. Your muscles tighten. You look into the darkness ahead and...and the next morning you have absolutely no idea what happened next. All you can remember is the sickening wash of fear as your mind was hijacked and held hostage by a nightmare.

70 percent of adults recognize that the **monsters aren't in our closets**—they're in our dreams.

Surprised? You shouldn't be. Believe it or not, it's not just our kids who have nightmares. Nearly 70 percent of adults do as well—with an amazing 30 percent of us reporting that these terrifying dreams jerk us out of sleep as often as once a month.

What Triggers a Nightmare?

Nightmares can be triggered by medications (for a list of drugs, see "Nightmare Meds" on page 192), oddball genes, degenerative neurological diseases like Alzheimer's, last night's tamales, traumatic events in the present, never-healed wounds from the past that a recent event has unmasked, and gut-level threats to health, safety, and the very sense of who you are.

Those who put a lid on expressing how they feel in response to stressful events during the day are likely to be taken for a ride by those emotions in the form of nightmares at night. And some, particularly people who are open and sensitive, may have a "thin" boundary between what's real and what's a dream—which means that their waking life is more than likely to stir up their night life and cause some pretty hairy dreams.

"A nightmare is a dysfunctional dream," explains Rosalind Cartwright, Ph.D., director of the sleep disorder service at Rush-Presbyterian–St. Luke's Medical Center in Chicago. Instead of integrating the day's events and feelings with older, stored memories and defusing negative emotions—which is what some researchers feel a dream is supposed to do—the emotions your brain is processing overload your circuits, prevent their integration into older memories, and jerk you from sleep.

If you're in a bad car accident, for example, you may not be able to process all the negative emotions the accident generates right away, says Dr. Cartwright. The fear and your sense of vulnerability and mortality are overwhelming. So you may have nightmares for a while as your mind keeps working away at integrating your feelings. Once it does, however, the nightmares go away.

As Dr. Cartwright eloquently writes in her book *Crisis Dreaming,* "Nightmares are a cry for resolution for finding a way to incorporate the terrible experience into our lives. Occasional nightmares are normal," she adds. "But not nightly, and not over and over again."

Some drugs—particularly antidepressants, barbiturates, sedatives, sleeping pills, beta-blockers, catacholaminergic agents, and amphetamines—can trigger nightmares. Surprisingly, however, so can the common antibiotic erythromycin and the over-the-counter anti-inflammatory naproxen. Other culprits include:

Betaxolol	*Nitrazepam*
Bisoprolol	*Paroxetine*
Bupropion	*Propranolol*
Carbachol	*Reserpine*
Donepezil	*Thioridazine*
Fluoxetine	*Triazolam*
Fluvoxamine	*Verapamil*
Levodopa	*Zolpidem tartrate extended-release*

When Nightmares Are a Sign of Danger

"Major depression usually wipes out dreaming altogether," says Dr. Cartwright. "Depressed people usually have no recall of dreaming, no dream content, no story. If they do, it's very short, very bland, with no feeling at all.

"As they recover from depression, however, their ability to dream comes back, and their dreams get more elaborate and full of emotion." Unfortunately, those recovering from depression can sometimes overshoot and be flooded with negative emotion.

"That's when suicides can occur," cautions Dr. Cartwright. So it's very important that anyone who is depressed report nightmares to their doctor immediately.

Banish Bad Dreams

Nightmares are a sign of overload. Check with a doctor, psychiatrist, or therapist if you're depressed, if they recur, or if you discover that your dreams are caused by distressing feelings from the past that have been triggered by current events.

Otherwise, here's how Rosalind Cartwright, Ph.D., director of the sleep disorder service at Rush-Presbyterian–St. Luke's Medical Center in Chicago and suggests you keep them at bay.

RECOGNIZE THAT THE DREAM IS BAD WHILE YOU'RE HAVING IT. This may sound impossible to do, but it's not. Simply resolve that you're going to do this before you fall asleep. It may take a few tries, but you'll get the hang of it.

IDENTIFY WHAT IN THE DREAM MAKES YOU FEEL BAD. What are the feelings or events involved?

STOP ANY BAD DREAM. Believe it or not, you can do it—often simply by recognizing that it's bad.

CHANGE THE ENDING. Turn what's negative into something positive. You may have to wake up to do it, but eventually you'll be able to tell yourself to write a better ending as you sleep.

KEEP A DREAM DIARY. Write down your dreams every morning. *All* your dreams, not just the nightmares. Then periodically review the ones that trouble you. Try to figure out why they're upsetting.

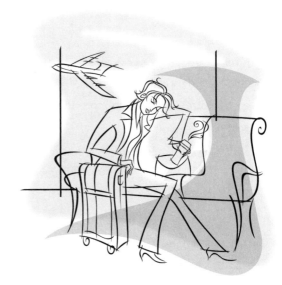

Jet Lag

Headed back from a well-deserved hiking vacation in Oregon, 38-year-old software executive Debbie Higgs climbed onto the huge Boeing 737 destined for New York, stowed a bag in the overhead bin, slid a laptop under her seat, and tucked a water bottle into the seat pocket in front of her. Then she sat down, buckled her seat belt, and turned on her iPod.

Jet lag affects **travelers** **physically,** **mentally,** and **emotionally.**

Only one thing was left to do before she closed her eyes and went to sleep: She shook a short-acting sleeping pill out of the bottle in her jacket pocket, popped it into her mouth, and washed it down with a swig of water.

Now she would sleep. She hoped.

Syncing into a New Time Zone

No one likes jet lag. We get off a flight feeling wrinkled and exhausted and then head into a day full of meetings or jump full swing into a vacation that had better be worth what we paid for it.

We never quite get up to speed the first day or two, and when our heads sink onto a pillow three, four, or five time zones away from home, we can't sleep. Or we sleep fitfully, tossing and turning, waking a half-dozen times.

In the morning all we want are directions to the nearest Starbucks.

"The problem," explains Lawrence J. Epstein, M.D., author of the *Harvard Medical School Guide to a Good Night's Sleep* and past president of the American Academy of Sleep Medicine, "is that your internal clock is out of sync with the external clock." It may be 7:00 A.M. according to all the clocks in New York when you land, for example, but if you're flying in from Portland like Debbie, your body's clock says it's 4:00 A.M. and you should be asleep.

Unfortunately, at the same time, light coming through your eyes into your brain is setting off your body's built-in chemical alarm clock, which is telling you to wake up.

The conflicting messages skating around in your brain produce that groggy hungover feeling that makes you sound about as bright and focused as Homer Simpson. That's

> "I frequently travel from London to New York and have to combat jet lag. I find that the only way to overcome it is to adapt to the time of my destination the minute I get on the plane. I can't listen to my body or else I'll never work through it. If it's an overnight flight, I try to sleep on the plane by putting on my special pair of battery-operated headphones that cut out all of the airplane noise. I refuse to leave home without them."
>
> —ZOË TOGHER

not a problem when you're on vacation, but it's certainly a serious issue if you're flying on company time and need to be at your best to make a sale or close a deal.

Fortunately, even though your whole sleep-wake system is pre-programmed by clock genes, it can still be manipulated by such factors as light, dark, temperature, a naturally occurring brain chemical, and medication.

One Woman's Story

SUZANNE PEACHTREE: Sleepless in San Diego

Suzanne Peachtree, a 43-year-old flight attendant who lives in San Diego, jumps into her car, smoothes down the skirt of her navy-blue uniform, and heads up the famously congested 5 freeway toward LAX—the huge international airport in Los Angeles.

It's a two-hour drive in the wee hours of the morning, but it's also Suzanne's passport to flights all over the world, entree to an ever-changing array of interesting people doing interesting things, and free air travel to vacation spots all around the globe.

The one drawback?

"It's very difficult to be perky at 3:00 A.M.," she admits. "I could get a full eight hours of sleep, work a civilized eight-hour day, and still feel like I want to die when my alarm clock goes off at 2:00 A.M."

Although she says she's gotten used to it after 18 years as a flight attendant, what's also difficult is the draggy feeling of jet lag and the flight schedules that play havoc on her sleep. "I could never give up coffee," she says with a shudder. "I don't care if it's bad for me. Some days it's the only thing that gets me out of bed."

Normally Suzanne flies 15 or 16 days a month. Each trip lasts from one to four days, and each workday lasts close to 16 hours. The variation in schedule plus the long workdays are enough to drive anyone's body clock nuts. But Suzanne is also constantly crossing and recrossing time zones from Hawaii to Europe. And it leaves her body thoroughly confused about when to wake and be alert or when to sleep and feel drowsy.

On a natural sleep schedule in her home time zone and with no alarm to wake her, Suzanne easily sleeps a straight nine hours. So she knows that's what her body really needs. She also knows that she can skate along on seven or eight hours' sleep when she works—so long as she gets no less than that.

"I would sacrifice almost anything for sleep," she says determinedly. "It's my number one priority." She uses heavy drapes to shut out light both at home and on the road, and she carries an eye mask and earplugs as a standard part of her travel kit. She often naps on a plane between flights—an old flight-attendant trick that explains why some of them look a bit rumpled prior to a late-night takeoff—and she has a standing prescription at the drugstore for "the hard stuff"—Ambien and Lunesta.

She also relies on melatonin. "It works like a charm," says Suzanne. "It helps me be sleepy whenever I'm not and need to be."

Reset Your Clock

Your body's internal clock is primarily set by your exposure to light and dark. Dark turns on production of the brain chemical melatonin, a naturally occurring compound that makes you sleepy; light turns production off so you are more alert.

When you travel, the light and dark cues change rapidly—confusing your internal clock and creating the hungover feeling of jet lag.

So if you want to avoid jet lag and its attendant insomnia, you need to gradually encourage your internal clock to get in sync with the light and dark cycles at your destination. That happens naturally over a 3- to 14-day period following your arrival. But for those of us who need to hit the ground running, researchers in recent years have found that one powerful way to reset your internal clock *before* you arrive is to alter your melatonin production schedule with the judicious use of a blue light specifically engineered to emit a particular wavelength, color, and intensity.

Scientists have known for some time that bright light can reset your body's clock. But until recently the only devices they had to do it with were huge, clunky boxes full of white fluorescent-style tubes that looked more as if they belonged backstage at a sleazy theater than in your home or office. Needless to say, not many people used them.

Now, however, powerful blue LED lights in plastic cases six inches square and an inch thick that slip into a tote or briefcase do the job. They're so small that some manufacturers have even incorporated blue lights into sun visors you can wear.

To give you some sense of what's involved in using blue light to prevent jet lag, Apollo Health, the company that made the lights used in most research studies, recommends that those traveling *east* wake up one hour early three days before they travel and sit near the blue-light box for 30 to 45 minutes each morning. You don't have to look directly at the light—you can set a blue-light box either beside your computer while you work or on the breakfast table while you eat. It does not emit UV radiation, and it's not harmful to children or pets. It does, however, bathe you in an electric blue light that makes you look like a member of off-Broadway's Blue Man Group. Any preschoolers in the house will love it.

A single session with a blue-light box will shift your body clock up to three time zones, according to the manufacturer. Then two days before travel, those traveling east should wake up *two* hours before their normal wake time and sit near the light a second time. On the day of departure, wake up *three* hours earlier than your normal wake time and sit near the light a third time.

Most flights from east to west take off in the morning. So when you arrive at your destination on the third day, wear sunglasses to make sure that no sunlight hits your eyes before 10:00 A.M. local time and messes up your light work. Even airport terminal lights can affect your body's time cues, so slip the sunglasses on as you enter the terminal.

When traveling west, use the light in the evening between 7:00 and 8:00 P.M. for 30 to 40 minutes two days before you travel. Use it again the night before you travel, starting an hour later. When you reach your destination, again use sunglasses—this time to protect yourself from any afternoon or evening light. Then ease your internal clock's transition back to home time by using your light each morning for a few days after you return.

If you're a regular road warrior, it may be worth your while to work with a sleep medicine specialist who can take into account the variables of your particular clock genes and scheduling priorities to develop a personal "light" prescription for shifting your internal clock before you travel.

Sleep across the Zones

There are 15 million of us who fly across multiple time zones every year, with 500,000 of us in the air at any given moment. And for those of us who fly more than a couple of time zones from home—particularly those who fly eastward around the globe—jet lag can be a serious challenge. It takes away our edge, makes us groggy, and disrupts our sleep. Here's how to be focused and alert during the day—and sound asleep at night.

ACCLIMATE. If you're going to be gone longer than a couple of days, begin acclimating your body to the new time zone by altering your eating schedule three days before your plane takes off.

If you're heading west to San Diego from Boston, for example, three days before you leave, eat an hour earlier each day. Flying from San Diego back to Boston? Help reverse the acclimation and get back on home time by eating an hour later each day for three days.

FLY A DAY EARLY. Some business travelers try to schedule multi–time zone meetings on a Monday so they can fly out Saturday afternoon or Sunday morning. That gives them a day or so to adjust their body's clock. It helps, travelers report. Employers don't appreciate the extra night's hotel bill, but since you're giving up your weekend, they usually fall in line. Unfortunately, nothing's going to square sacrificing yet another work weekend to your family.

CHUG. Stay hydrated with bottled water. Avoid alcohol and anything caffeinated during your flight. Both can dehydrate your body, mess up your internal clock, and exaggerate jet lag symptoms.

FLY BUSINESS OR FIRST CLASS. If you're flying overnight and need to hit the ground running in the morning, book a business or first-class seat so you can get some sleep. Sitting upright in a narrower economy seat with no legroom, your body generates adrenaline-like substances to keep blood flowing up to your brain. The adrenaline keeps you from sleeping, and if you do doze off, it keeps you from dropping into a restorative sleep. On the other hand, lying in a flatter position with the legroom accorded to first-class and business-class seating prevents the problem altogether, and you can arrive at your destination rested, focused, and ready to go.

HIT THE LINGUINE. Or any other carb-dense food at dinner on the night before your flight. Scientists have been arguing for some time about whether or not this decreases jet lag and increases your potential for normal sleep, but recent research on clock genes has uncovered subtle effects that indicate carbs boost your ability to sleep—particularly when you fly westward. No one's quite figured out how they help, but they do know that carbs provide your brain with a source of tryptophan from which it can make the sleep-inducing neurotransmitter serotonin.

REFRIGERATE. If you're flying during what would be night hours at your destination, try to get some sleep on the plane. Use earplugs to eliminate noise, an eyeshade to kill the light, and turn the air-conditioning valve on high. A third cue your body uses to set its internal clock is temperature. A lower temperature lowers your body's core temperature and signals it's time for sleep. A higher temperature raises your body's core temperature and signals that it's time to wake. To keep from getting too chilled, bring along one of those silk blanket-and-pillow sets that are sold through airline and online travel catalogs.

AVOID AIRLINE FOOD. A fourth cue your body uses to set its internal clock is food. Since airline food is served onboard according to the time at your home base, eating it can sabotage efforts to reset your clock to the time zone to which you're traveling.

CONSIDER THE MEDICAL OPTION. Short-acting sleeping pills can help you sleep through an overnight flight. They can also help you sleep during the first couple of nights at your destination. That said, keep in mind that if a sleeping pill is taken just a little later than it should be on local time, it can exacerbate the effects of jet lag. Even worse, if the drug lasts longer than the flight, you'll arrive drowsy at your destination—that's not good if you have to drive or negotiate local transportation home.

CONSIDER MELATONIN. Yes, it's available as an over-the-counter medication and you don't need a prescription. But since it has the ability to really mess with your brain chemicals, consult with a doctor anyway—especially if you're taking another medication.

Studies indicate that supplemental melatonin will make you sleepy. It's not as strong as a sleeping pill, but it directly affects your body's internal clock and nudges it toward sleep.

Generally, sleep specialists seem to recommend that if you're heading east, you should consider taking one 3- to 5-milligram capsule between 6:00 and 7:00 P.M. on the day you fly out. Take a second capsule after you've arrived at the local bedtime.

If you do take melatonin, however, think about taking a cab to your hotel and picking up a rental car at the hotel rather than the airport. You may be too drowsy to drive safely.

If you're headed west, take a single melatonin capsule just before bed at your destination. Do not take it before your flight.

Two caveats: One, because it's not reviewed by the FDA, over-the-counter melatonin can come in vastly differing qualities. So buy a well-known brand from a company that guarantees its products. Two, the safety profile of melatonin has not been seriously investigated. It is not, experts agree, for long-term use until studies verifying its safety over the long haul have been done. So don't think it's something you can continue to use at home on a regular basis.

HAVE THE EGGS BENEDICT. A protein-rich meal the morning after you arrive will give your brain what it needs to produce neurochemicals to increase your alertness throughout the day.

STAY ON HOME TIME. If you're going to be away from home for only a couple of days, stay on the same eating and sleeping schedule while you're away as you would at home. If you normally have dinner in Atlanta at 8:00 P.M. for instance, when you fly to Los Angeles for two days of business meetings, have dinner at 5:00 P.M. You'll not only avoid that dragged-around-by-your-hair jet-lagged feeling, you also won't have trouble getting a good table at the restaurant of your choice.

OR SWITCH IMMEDIATELY. If you're away for more than just a couple of days, don't just set your watch to local time when you arrive—help reset your internal clock by eating, going to bed, and waking at the local time as well.

BRING YOUR WORKOUT GEAR. Most hotels have exercise rooms and lap pools. Schedule a 30-minute workout each day you're on the road. You'll feel and sleep better.

WATCH OUT FOR FUZZ BRAIN. Avoid driving long distances and making critical decisions for the first 24 hours after you arrive. If you're the least bit fuzzed by jet lag, your ability to think and react will be impaired.

MAKE IT DARK AND COLD. Yeah, the view from your hotel-room window is superb. But use those heavy room-darkening shades to shut out light during the hours you plan to sleep. Also, lower the room's temperature. Remember, manipulating light and temperature manipulates your body's clock and gives it a clear mandate to sleep.

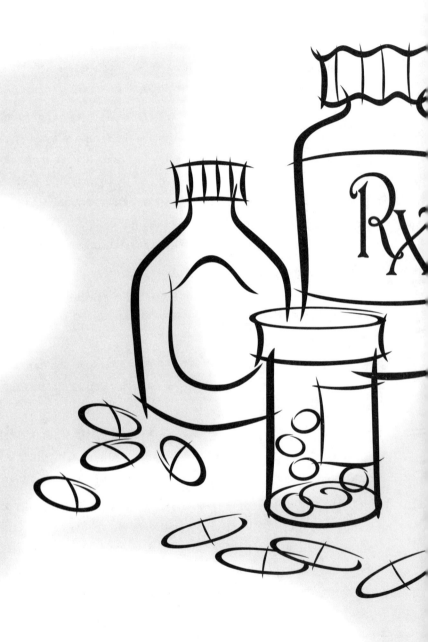

Part IV

The New Meds
Are They Better than the Old?

A Quick Fix

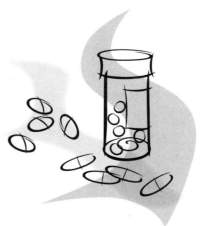

Sleeping pills have become a way of life for an amazing number of women trying to survive and compete in today's world. Whether they're overworked short-order cooks with a family of five to support, Bluetooth-enabled businesswomen with the responsibility for multimillion-dollar companies, critical-care nurses in high-tech

29 percent of women take a sleeping pill at least **several nights a week.**

hospitals with patients' lives on the line, or graphic artists working an extra shift at the local grocery store to put their kids through college, the fact is that women are working harder than they ever have before. Unfortunately, sleep is one of those things that often doesn't get with the program.

The trouble is, since there are so many sleep aids available—benzodiazepines, non-benzodiazepines, melatonin agonists, and even antidepressants and antihistamines—each with its own level of potency and side effects, it's important to find which one is best for you.

Finding the "True Fix"

"Sleep meds can be quite beneficial," says Lawrence J. Epstein, M.D., recent president of the American Academy of Sleep Medicine, author of *The Harvard Medical School Guide to a Good Night's Sleep*, and medical director of the Harvard-affiliated Sleep Health*Centers*. "They tend to be most helpful in people with short-term problems."

Your mother dies, you get fired from a job, you're going through a nasty divorce—that's where they can help. Just for a night or two until you get on a more even keel. Unfortunately, that's not how most of us use them. Studies show that most people who take sleeping pills take them for two years. And a full third take them for five.

"People want a quick fix rather than a true fix," explains Dr. Epstein. Sleep hygiene strategies, like getting to bed at the same time every night, getting up at the same time every day, and only staying in bed

OVER-THE-COUNTER SLEEP MEDS

Histamines, a chemical naturally produced by the body in response to an allergen, promote alertness. *Anti*histamines, a chemical produced by a pharmaceutical company to reduce allergy symptoms, encourages drowsiness. Some people turn to antihistamines to promote sleep. However, antihistamines can cause additional side effects, such as dizziness, stomach problems, nausea, and a lack of muscle coordination. After the fourth day of use, the body ignores the call to drowse.

while you're asleep are powerful. And studies show that cognitive behavioral therapy (CBT) is just as effective as a pill—plus its effects last a lot longer. (For more information see "Does Online Sleep Therapy Work?" beginning on page 30.)

"But CBT needs a commitment," says Dr. Epstein. To a series of meetings. To a series of lifestyle changes. And people don't want to do either.

"The hardest thing in medicine is to get someone to make a lifestyle change," he admits ruefully. But the thing is, you have to do it. "If no one else is going to bed or everyone else is going out dancing, you have to say, 'My biological clock says I need to sleep.'"

> In a study of 277 teens, researchers found that 14.9 percent of kids ages 13 to 17 have used sleep meds at least once.

How to Use Sleep Meds Effectively

The four most important things for you—and your doctor—to know about a sleep medication is how quickly it starts to work, how long it lasts, what side effects it has, and whether or not it interacts with any other medication you may be taking.

If you have trouble *falling* asleep, any medication you use should work fast and dissipate quickly, says Dr. Epstein. If you have trouble *staying* asleep or *waking* at the crack of dawn, any medication you use should last through the night, but not so long that you wake up groggy.

Benzodiazepines. That said, the sleep meds that are the most thoroughly tested and are the best tolerated belong to a family of chemicals called benzodiazepines, says Dr. Epstein. They basically knock you out, and some also reduce anxiety and seizures.

Non-benzodiazepines. A second group of sleep meds are the non-benzodiazepines. They're the new kids on the block that are advertised every third minute on American television—Ambien, Lunesta, and Sonata. They work quickly to get you to sleep and don't last very long.

Melatonin. A third group, the newest, are the melatonin agonists. Only one is FDA-approved for sale in the United States so far, but more are on the way. The one that's been approved—Rozerem—works quickly, doesn't hang around, and the sedating effect is pretty mild. Essentially, it allows you to shift your biological clock. There's also over-the-counter melatonin, adds Dr. Epstein, but there's little information about its safety. Since it's an over-the-counter drug, its effectiveness and quality are not regulated by the FDA.

Antidepressants and Antihistamines

So which meds are the most popular? Although these medications offer us a variety of options, the fact is that the class of drugs most often prescribed for insomnia are antidepressants, says Dr. Epstein. None of them have been studied as a treatment for insomnia, so no one has any idea how effective they are for that purpose. And since antidepressants can already be prescribed for other conditions, he adds, the companies that manufacture them aren't likely to bankroll studies to find out.

But there's an arguably even more popular sleep medication—over-the-counter antihistamines. Nearly 25 percent of those of us with insomnia use old drugs like Benadryl to make ourselves drowsy. "They change the level of histamine in the brain, which can make people sleepy," says Dr. Epstein. "There's no data on their effectiveness, however, and they probably have a higher side-effect profile than benzodiazepines. Men with prostate problems shouldn't take them."

According to Dr. Epstein, an over-the-counter antihistamine is potentially more dangerous than a benzodiazepene. And they only work for about four nights in a row," he says.

Clearly, sleep medications should be taken only after a thoughtful consultation with your physician. But you may also want to discuss a new study from the Finnish Institute of Occupational Health in Helsinki. Researchers there followed 21,268 twins for 22 years. They found that "frequent" use of sleep medications increased the risk of death in women by 39 percent. Further research is necessary to find out why.

A comparison of old and new sleep medications reveals that newer

ANTIDEPRESSANTS USED FOR SLEEP

Antidepressants are not approved by the FDA or Health Canada to treat insomnia, nor are there studies or convincing evidence to support their use. Nevertheless, antidepressants are the medication most likely to be prescribed by your doctor when you ask for "something to help me sleep." All have significant side effects such as headache, nausea, anxiety, and weight gain. Common antidepressants include:

Brand Name	Generic Name
Elavil	amitriptyline
Celexa	citalopram
Sinequan	doxepin
Prozac	fluoxetine
Remeron	mirtazapine
Paxil	paroxetine
Zoloft	saertraline
Desyrel	trazodone

drugs, like zolpidem, eszopiclone, ramelteon, and zaleplon, reduce the time it takes to get to sleep between 12 and 20 minutes. Older drugs, like Dalmane, Halcion and Restoril, reduce the time it takes from between 11 and 23 minutes.

Those who took the new sleep medications got between 8 and 25 minutes more sleep each night. Those who took the older drugs got between 12 and 40 minutes more sleep.

Which is the best drug for you? Only you and your doctor know for sure.

SLEEP MEDICATIONS

The following sleep aids reduce the time it takes for someone to fall asleep. The table shows how much faster you're able to get to sleep after taking these aids, as well as the number of minutes on average your "waking period" is reduced by in the middle of the night. It's interesting to compare the effects of these medications with cognitive behavioral therapy (see "Work

New Sleep Meds

Brand Name	Generic Name*	How Much Faster It Takes to Get to Sleep (minutes)	Amount of Time Waking Period Is Reduced (minutes)	Common Side Effects
Ambien	zolpidem	12.8	8.5	Daytime drowsiness, headache, nausea, dizziness, grogginess
Lunesta	eszopiclone	16.7	25.8	Daytime drowsiness, headache, nausea, dizziness, grogginess
Rozerem	ramelteon	15	11	Dizziness, may exacerbate symptoms of depression
Sonata	zaleplon	20.1	—	Daytime drowsiness, headache, nausea, dizziness, grogginess

May be sold under a different name, depending on the country where you live.

with a Cognitive Behavioral Therapist" on page 79). Studies show that those who use cognitive behavioral therapy get to sleep about 35 minutes faster. And it reduces the time you spend awake in the middle of the night by about 38 minutes.

Old Sleep Meds

Brand Name	Generic Name	How Much Faster It Takes to Get to Sleep (minutes)	Amount of Time Waking Period Is Reduced (minutes)	Common Side Effects
Dalmane	flurazepam	23.1	12.4	Daytime drowsiness, unsteadiness, light-headedness, headache
Halcion	triazolam	19.7	40.0	Daytime drowsiness, unsteadiness, light-headedness, headache
Restoril	temazepam	11.6	23.7	Daytime drowsiness, unsteadiness, light-headedness, headache

Sources:
1. Harvard Medical School. *Guide to a Good Night's Sleep,* 2007.

2. Ramakrishnan, K. *American Family Physician,* August 2007.

3. Roth, T. et al. *Sleep Med,* June 2006.

4. Zammit G. et al. *Journal of Sleep Medicine,* August 2007.

Resources
Sleep Centers

"Sleep is the new bottled water!" crowed the *New York Times* not long ago—and they were absolutely right.

As each of us begins to recognize the effects of a globalized economy with 24/7 demands on our sleep—and as research reveals the effects of sleep on our performance, health, happiness, waistline, and longevity—sleep is trending up, and sleep centers and sleep labs are popping up all across the globe.

"The good news is that sleep medicine is increasingly included in medical school curricula," says Hrayr P. Attarian, M.D., director of the University of Vermont's regional sleep center and editor of the textbook *Sleep Disorders in Women*. "The bad news is that some entrepreneurial people are trying to make money off sleep. It's become a very lucrative field. Businessmen, lawyers, and accountants are starting their own sleep labs, loosely associated with a doctor." Unfortunately, he adds, "most are not accredited."

To make sure you get physicians who are actually trained in sleep medicine, steer clear of freestanding centers headed by people other than physicians, advises Dr. Attarian. Instead, look for a center accredited by the American Academy of Sleep Medicine.

To give you a place to start, we've listed a number of accredited centers on the following pages. We've also included telephone numbers, Web sites, and street addresses. So all you have to do is pick up your phone or mouse—and help is at your fingertips. You can also check out www.sleepcenters.org, which adds new centers to their Web site as they're accredited by the academy.

We've also included a list of sleep centers across Canada, Australia, New Zealand, and the United Kingdom. Please note that there is no accrediting agency in these countries; these centers have not been certified by a national professional organization. Again, look for centers run by doctors—not the neighborhood investment counselor.

In the United States

ALABAMA

Crestwood Center for Sleep Disorders
Crestwood Medical Center
250 Chateau Drive
Suite 235
Huntsville, AL 35801
(256) 880-4710
www.crestwoodmedcenter.com

Decatur General Sleep Disorders Center
Decatur General Hospital
1201 7th Street SE
Decatur, AL 35601
(256) 341-2915
www.decaturgeneral.org

Jackson Sleep Disorders Center
Jackson Hospital
1722 Pine Street
Suite 300
Montgomery, AL 36106
(334) 293-8168
medsouthinc.net

Sleep Disorders Center at HealthSouth Medical Center
1201 11th Avenue S
Birmingham, AL 35205
(205) 930-8295

ARIZONA

Mayo Clinic Hospital Sleep Disorders Center
Mayo Clinic Hospital
5777 East Mayo Boulevard
Phoenix, AZ 85054
(480) 342-1018
www.mayoclinic.com

Scottsdale Sleep Center
9767 N. 91st Street
Suite 104
Scottsdale, AZ 85258
(480) 767-8811
www.scottsdalesleepcenter.com

ARKANSAS

Arkansas Center for Sleep Medicine
500 South University Avenue
Suite 506
Little Rock, AR 72205
(501) 661-9191
www.arsleep.com

WRMC Sleep Disorders Center
Washington Regional Medical Center
1708 Joyce Street
Fayetteville, AR 72703
(479) 527-0471
www.wregional.com

CALIFORNIA

Clinical Monitoring Center, Inc.
Sleep Disorders Center
20410 Town Center Lane
Suite F-150
Cupertino, CA 95014
(408) 523-3460
www.sleepscape.com

Scripps Clinic Sleep Center
10666 N. Torrey Pines Road
La Jolla, CA 92037
(858) 554-8845
www.scrippsclinic.com

Sleep Disorders Center
Community Hospital of the Monterey Peninsula
2 Upper Ragsdale Drive
Building D, Suite 220
Monterey, CA 93940
(831) 649-7210
www.chomp.org

Southern California Sleep Disorders Specialists
947 S. Anaheim Boulevard
Suite 210
Anaheim, CA 92805
(714) 491-1159
www.sleepcenters.org/socalsleep

UCDHS Sleep Disorders Center
University of California, Davis
   Medical Center
2315 Stockton Boulevard
Room 5308
Sacramento, CA 95817
(916) 734-0256

UCSF Sleep Disorders Center
University of California San Francisco
   Medical Center
1600 Divisadero Street
San Francisco, CA 94115
(415) 885-7886
www.mountzion.ucsfmedicalcenter.org/
   sleep_center/

COLORADO
Parkview Medical Center Sleep Center
400 W. Sixteenth Street
Pueblo, CO 81003
(719) 584-4976
www.parkviewmc.com/pmc.nsf/View/
   SleepCenterDisorders

**Sleep Center at National Jewish
   Medical and Research Center**
1400 Jackson Street
Suite A200
Denver, CO 80206
(303) 270-2708
www.nationaljewish.org

Sleep Disorders Center
Penrose/St. Francis Health Center
825 E. Pikes Peak Avenue
Colorado Springs, CO 80903
(719) 776-8868
www.penrosestfrancis.org

CONNECTICUT
**The Center for Sleep Medicine at
   Bridgeport Hospital**
267 Grant Street
West Tower 6
Bridgeport, CT 06610
(203) 384-3817
www.bridgeporthospital.org/CenterSleepMedicine

**Danbury Hospital Sleep
   Disorders Center**
Danbury Hospital
24 Hospital Avenue
Danbury, CT 06810
(203) 731-8033
www.danhosp.org

Yale Sleep Medicine
40 Tempe Street
New Haven, CT 06510
(203) 764-6788
www.info.med.yale.edu/intmed/sleep/

DISTRICT OF COLUMBIA
Sleep Disorders Center
Georgetown University Medical Center
3800 Reservoir Road NW
5th Floor, Main Building, Room 5411
Washington, DC 20007
(202) 444-3610
http://www.georgetownuniversityhospital.org/
   body.cfm?id=263

The Sleep Disorders Center
The George Washington University Hospital
900 23rd Street NW
4th Floor
Washington, DC 20037
(202) 715-4000

DELAWARE
Sleep Disorders Center
Christiana Care Health Services
774 Christiana Road
Suite 103
Newark, DE 19713
(302) 623-0650
www.christianacare.org

Sleep Disorders Center at Bayhealth
Bayhealth Medical Center
540 S. Governors Avenue
Suite 101C
Dover, DE 19901
(302) 744-7152

FLORIDA

Boca Raton Sleep Disorders Center
660 Glades Road
Suite 220
Boca Raton, FL 33431-6466
(561) 750-9881

Florida Hospital Sleep Disorders Center at Orlando
Florida Hospital Orlando
601 E. Rollins Street
Orlando, FL 32803
(407) 303-1558
www.flhosp.org/services/sleepdisorders/

Sleepcare Diagnostics–Sarasota
6003 Honore Avenue
Suite 101
Sarasota, FL 34238
(941) 927-9686
www.snorenomore.com/Sarasota

Sleep Disorders Center
Broward General Medical Center
1600 S. Andrews Avenue
Fort Lauderdale, FL 33316
(954) 355-5532
www.browardhealth.org

Sleep Disorders Center
Mayo Clinic Jacksonville
4500 San Pablo Road
Jacksonville, FL 32224
(904) 953-7287
www.mayoclinic.org/sleepdisorders-jax/

The Sleep Disorders Center
Cedars Medical Center
1400 NW 12th Avenue
Miami, FL 33136
(305) 325-4518
www.cedars.com

Sleep Disorders Center Florida
1355 37th Street
Suite 302
Vero Beach, FL 32960
(772) 770-4888
www.sleepcenters.org/sleepdisordersflorida

GEORGIA

Atlanta Center for Sleep Disorders
Atlanta Medical Center
303 Parkway Drive, NE
Box 44
Atlanta, GA 30312
(404) 265-3733
www.atlantamedcenter.com

MCG Sleep Disorders Center
Medical College of Georgia Health, Inc.
(MCGHI)
1120 15th Street
Room BT4720
Augusta, GA 30912
(706) 721-0791
www.mcghealth.org/health_services/
sleep_center/index.html

Sleep Disorders Center
Children's Healthcare of Atlanta at
Scottish Rite
1001 Johnson Ferry Road, NE
Atlanta, GA 30342
(404) 250-2096

Sleep Disorders Center of Georgia
5505 Peachtree Dunwoody Road
Suite 380
Atlanta, GA 30342
(404) 257-0080
www.sleepsciences.com

Sleep Disorders Center
DeKalb Medical Center
2701 N. Decatur Road
Decatur, GA 30033
(404) 501-5927
www.dekalbmedicalcenter.org

Sleep Disorders Center
Memorial Health University Medical Center
4700 Waters Avenue
Savannah, GA 31403
(912) 350-8327
www.memorialhealth.com

HAWAII
Sleep Disorders Center of the Pacific
Straub Clinic & Hospital
888 South King Street
Honolulu, HI 96813
(808) 522-4448
www.hawaiipacifichealth.org/

Sleep Disorders Laboratory
North Hawaii Community Hospital
67-1125 Mamalahoa Highway
Kamuela, HI 96743
(808) 881-4876
www.northhawaiicommunityhospital.org

The Sleep Lab, A Sleep Related Breathing Disorders Laboratory
46-001 Kamehameha Hwy #314
Kaneohe, HI 96744
(808) 234-0033

IDAHO
Idaho Sleep Disorders Center–Boise
St. Luke's Regional Medical Center
190 E. Bannock Street
Boise, ID 83712
www.ucomparehealthcare.com/hospital/
    Idaho/St_Lukes_Regional_Medical_
    Center.html

Idaho Sleep Disorders Center– Meridian
St. Luke's Meridian Medical Center
520 S. Eagle Road
Meridian, ID 83642
(208) 706-5380
www.stlukesonline.org

St. Joseph Regional Medical Center Sleep Center
St. Joseph Regional Medical Center
415 6th Street
Lewiston, ID 83501
(208) 799-5484
www.sjrmc.org/services.htm

Southeast Idaho Sleep Disorders Center
Portineuf Medical Center
651 Memorial Drive
Pocatello, ID 83201
(208) 239-2631

ILLINOIS
The Center for Sleep Medicine
680 N. Lake Shore Drive
Suite 1210
Chicago, IL 60611
(312) 587-3765
www.sleepmedcenter.com

Evanston Hospital Sleep Disorders Center
Evanston Northwestern Healthcare
2650 Ridge Avenue
Evanston, IL 60201
(847) 570-2567
www.enh.org/clinicalservices/
    neurosciences/programs

Provena Sleep Disorder Center
Provena Saint Joseph Medical Center
300 Barney Drive
Suite C
Joliet, IL 60435
(815) 744-7762
www.provenasaintjoe.org

Sleep Disorders Center
Northwest Community Hospital
901 W. Kirchoff Road
Arlington Heights, IL 60005
(847) 618-3190
www.nch.org

Sleep Disorders Center
The University of Chicago Hospitals
5841 S. Maryland Avenue
Chicago, IL 60637
(773) 702-5871
www.uchospitals.edu/specialties/
    pulmonary/sleep-disorders/

INDIANA

Community Health Network
Sleep/Wake Disorders Center South
1402 E. Country Line Road
Indianapolis, IN 46227
(317) 887-7079
www.ecommunity.com/sleep/

Memorial Sleep Disorders Center
53990 Carmichael Drive
Suite 150
South Bend, IN 46635
(574) 247-1850
http://www.qualityoflife.org/services/sleep-disorders/

St. Joseph Sleep Disorders Center
St. Joseph Medical Center
700 Broadway
Fort Wayne, IN 46802
(260) 425-3552
www.lutheranhealthnetwork.com

Sleep Disorders Center
St. Vincent Hospital & Health Services
8401 Harcourt Road
Indianapolis, IN 46260
(317) 338-2152
www.stvincent.org

IOWA

Eastern Iowa Sleep Center
600 Seventh St. SE
Cedar Rapids, IA 52401
(319) 362-4433
www.eisleep.com

Iowa Sleep Disorders Center
4080 Westown Parkway
Des Moines, IA 50266
(515) 225-0188
www.iowasleep.com

Sleep Disorders Center
University of Iowa Hospitals and Clinics
200 Hawkins Drive
Iowa City, IA 52242
(319) 356-3813

KANSAS

KU Department of Neurology Sleep Medicine Clinic
3901 Rainbow Boulevard
Kansas City, KS 66160
(913) 588-5273

Olathe Medical Center Sleep Disorders Center
Olathe Medical Center, Inc.
20333 W. 151st Street
Olathe, KS 66061
(913) 791-4282
www.home.ohsi.com/

St. Catherine Hospital Neurodiagnostic & Sleep Disorders Center
St. Catherine Hospital
401 E. Spruce
Garden City, KS 67846
(620) 272-2420

KENTUCKY

Sleep Diagnostics Center
Greenview Regional Hospital
1801 Ashley Circle
Bowling Green, KY 42104
(270) 793-2175

The Sleep Disorders Center
St. Luke Hospital West
7380 Turfway Road
Florence, KY 41042
(859) 962-5347
www.drscheer.go.to

Sleep Disorders Center of Lexington
3121 Wall Street
Suite 200
Lexington, KY 40513
(859) 223-9990
www.sleepdisorderscenter.net

LOUISIANA

Comprehensive Sleep
Medicine Center
Tulane University Medical Center
1415 Tulane Avenue
7th Floor
New Orleans, LA 70112
(504) 988-1657

Sleep Disorder Center of Louisiana
4820 Lake Street
Lake Charles, LA 70605
(337) 310-7378

Sleep Disorders Center
Ochsner Health Center–Baton Rouge
9001 Summa Avenue
Baton Rouge, LA 70809
(225) 761-5200
www.ochsner.org

MAINE

Maine Sleep Institute
Maine Medical Center
930 Congress Street
Portland, ME 04102
(207) 662-4535
www.mmc.org

Sleep Center of Maine
Eastern Maine Medical Center
489 State Street
P.O. Box 404
Bangor, ME 04402-0404
(207) 973-5892
www.emmc.org

MARYLAND

Johns Hopkins University Sleep
Disorders Center
Johns Hopkins Bayview Medical Center
5501 Hopkins Bayview Circle
Asthma & Allergy Building, Room 4B50
Baltimore, MD 21224
(410) 550-2530
www.hopkinsbayview.org/

Sinai Hospital Sleep Disorders Center
Sinai Hospital
2401 W. Belvedere Avenue
Baltimore, MD 21215
(410) 601-9523

Sleep Disorders Center at
Memorial Hospital
Memorial Hospital at Easton
219 S. Washington Street
Easton, MD 21601
(410) 822-1000

MASSACHUSETTS

The Center for Sleep Diagnostics
Neurocare, Inc.
70 Wells Avenue
Suite #101
Newton, MA 02459
(617) 796-7766
www.neurocareinc.com

New England Medical Center
Center for Sleep Medicine
750 Washington Street
Boston, MA 02111
(617) 636-7689
www.nemc.org/home/departments/adult/
   pulmcrit.htm

MICHIGAN

Genesys Sleep Disorders Center
Genesys Regional Medical Center
Genesys West Flint Campus
3921 Beecher Road
Flint, MI 48532-3699
(810) 762-4676
www.genesys.org

Sleep-Wake Disorders Center
John D. Dingell VA Medical Center
Neurology Section 11M-NEU
4646 John R. Street
Detroit, MI 48201
(313) 576-3663

University of Michigan Sleep Disorders Center
University of Michigan Hospitals
1500 E. Medical Center Drive
C728 Med Inn Building
Ann Arbor, MI 48109-0845
(734) 647-9068
www.med.umich.edu/neuro/sleeplab/

MINNESOTA
Duluth Regional Sleep Disorders Center
St. Mary's Medical Center
407 E. Third Street
Duluth, MN 55805
(218) 786-4692
www.stmarysduluth.org/

Minnesota Regional Sleep Disorders Center
Hennepin County Medical Center
701 Park Avenue
Minneapolis, MN 55415
(612) 873-6201
www.hcmc.org

Minnesota Sleep Institute
High Pointe Health Campus Sleep Disorders Center
High Pointe Health Campus
8650 Hudson Boulevard
Lake Elmo, MN 55042
(651) 501-2035

MISSISSIPPI
Delta Regional Medical Center Sleep Center
Delta Regional Medical Center
300 S. Washington Avenue
Greenville, MS 38701
(662) 725-1118
www.tkdh.com

University of Mississippi Sleep Disorders Center
University of Mississippi Medical Center
2500 N. State Street
Box 153
Jackson, MS 39216
(601) 984-4820
www.psych.umc.edu/

MISSOURI
Clayton Sleep Institute
2531 S. Big Bend Boulevard
Suite 2
Saint Louis, MO 63143
(314) 645-5855
www.claytoninstitute.com

Sleep Disorders Center at St. Luke's Hospital
4301 Wornall Road
Kansas City, MO 64111
(816) 932-3382
www.saintlukeshealthsystem.org/slhs/
    Locations/Center_for_Health_
    Enhancement

University of Missouri Sleep Disorders Center
University of Missouri Hospital/University of Missouri Health Care
1 Hospital Drive
C2020, Diagnostic Center
Columbia, MO 65212
(573) 884-7533
www.muhealth.org/~hospital/
    sleepcenter.shtml

MONTANA
Billings Clinic Sleep Disorders Center
Billings Clinic
2800 8th Avenue N
Billings, MT 59101-7000
(406) 238-2885
www.billingsclinic.org

**Bozeman Deaconess Sleep
Disorders Center**
Bozeman Deaconess Hospital
915 Highland Boulevard
Bozeman, MT 59715
(406) 585-5058
www.bozemandeaconess.org

St. Patrick Hospital Sleep Center
St. Patrick Hospital
500 W. Broadway
Missoula, MT 59802
(406) 329-5650
www.saintpatrick.org

NEBRASKA
Bryan LGH Center for Sleep Medicine
2300 S. 16th Street
Lincoln, NE 68502
(402) 481-9646
www.bryanlgh.org/go/medical-
services/sleep-medicine

**Methodist Hospital Sleep
Disorders Center**
Methodist Healthwest
16120 W. Dodge Road
Omaha, NE 68118
(402) 354-0825

NEVADA
Desert Sleep Disorders Center
Nevada Lung Center
9820 W. Sunset Road
Suite 312
Las Vegas, NV 89148
(702) 737-1409

**Pulmonary Medicine Associates
Sleep Center**
601 S. Arlington Avenue
Reno, NV 89503
(775) 329-1727
www.pmareno.com

NEW HAMPSHIRE
Center for Sleep Evaluation
Elliot Hospital
1 Elliot Way
Manchester, NH 03103-3599
(603) 663-6680
www.elliothospital.org/services

**Dartmouth-Hitchcock Sleep
Disorders Center**
Dartmouth-Hitchcock Medical Center
1 Medical Center Drive
Lebanon, NH 03756
(603) 650-7534

Sleep Center at Concord Hospital
Concord Hospital
250 Pleasant Street
Concord, NH 03301
(603) 228-7022

NEW JERSEY
Center for Sleep Disorders
Community Medical Center
67 Route 37
Riverwood I
Toms River, NJ 08755
(732) 557-2798
www.saintbarnabas.com/hospitals/
community_medical/services/
sleepdisorders.html

Institute for Sleep/Wake Disorders
Hackensack University Medical Center
30 Prospect Avenue
Hackensack, NJ 07601
(201) 996-3732
www.humc.net

**Sleep Disorder Center of Morristown
Memorial Hospital**
Morristown Memorial Hospital
95 Mount Kemble Avenue
Morristown, NJ 07962
(973) 971-4567
www.atlantichealth.org

Virtua/Memorial Hospital of
   Burlington County/Cherry Hill
457 Haddonfield Road
Liberty View Building, Suite 520
Cherry Hill, NJ 08002
(800) 753-3779
www.sleepcarecenter.com

NEW MEXICO

**St. Vincent Regional Medical Center:
   Sleep Disorders Center**
455 St. Michaels Drive
Santa Fe, NM 87505
(505) 820-5363
www.stvin.org/applications/specialties/

UNMH Sleep Disorders Center
The University of New Mexico
   Health Sciences Center
1101 Medical Arts Avenue, NE
Building 2
Albuquerque, NM 87102
(505) 272-6021
www.hospitals.unm.edu/SDC/

NEW YORK

**Bassett Healthcare Sleep
   Disorders Center**
1 Atwell Road
Cooperstown, NY 13326
(607) 547-6306
www.bassethealthcare.org

**Center for Sleep Disorders Medicine
   & Research**
New York Methodist Hospital
506 Sixth Street
Brooklyn, NY 11215
(718) 780-3017

St. Peter's Sleep Center
St. Peter's Hospital
Pine West Plaza #1
Washington Avenue Extension
Albany, NY 12205
(518) 464-9999
www.stpetershealthcare.org

**Sleep Disorders Center at Montefiore
   Medical Center**
111 E. 210th Street
Bronx, NY 10583
(718) 920-4841
www.cloud9.net/~thorpy/mmc/

NORTH CAROLINA

Duke Sleep Disorders Center
Duke University Medical Center
2800 Campus Walk Avenue
Durham, NC 27705
(919) 684-3196
www.dukehealth.org

The Sleep Center at SouthPark
Charlotte Eye Ear Nose and Throat
   Associates, P.A.
6300 Morrison Boulevard
Suite 667
Charlotte, NC 28211
(704) 295-3000
www.goodsenses.com

**University of North Carolina Sleep
   Disorders Center**
University of North Carolina Hospitals
101 Manning Drive
Chapel Hill, NC 27514
(919) 966-3294

NORTH DAKOTA

MeritCare Sleep Disorders Center
MeritCare Health System
1717 S. University Drive
West Complex A–3rd Floor
Fargo, ND 58103
(701) 280-4600

North Dakota Center for Sleep
A Division of PDS
4152 30th Avenue S
Suite #103
Fargo, ND 58104
(701) 356-3000
www.ndsleep.com

OHIO

Akron General Medical Center Sleep Disorders Center
Akron General Medical Center
400 Wabash Avenue
Akron, OH 44307
(330) 344-6751
www.akrongeneral.org

Grant Medical Center Sleep Disorders Center
Grant Medical Center
285 E. State Street
Suite 425
Columbus, OH 43215
(614) 566-9895

Kettering Hospital Sleep Disorders Center
45 W. Grand Avenue
Dayton, OH
(937) 395-8805

Sleep Management Institute–Red Bank
4460 Red Bank Highway #230
Cincinnati, OH 45227
(513) 977-8882
www.sleepmanagement.md

West Region Sleep Center
15805 Puritas Avenue
Cleveland, OH 44135
(216) 267-5933

OKLAHOMA

Integris Sleep Disorders Center of Oklahoma
Baptist Medical Center
3300 Northwest Expressway
Oklahoma City, OK 73112
(405) 951-8333
www.integris-health.com

Sleep Disorders Center at St. Francis Hospital
6585 South Yale Avenue
Suite 650
Tulsa, OK 74136
(918) 502-6000
www.saintfrancis.com

OREGON

High Desert Sleep Disorders Center
St. Charles Medical Center
2042 Williamson Court
Bend, OR 97701
(541) 383-6905
www.scmc.org/services_listing.html

Legacy Sleep Disorders Center
Legacy Good Samaritan Hospital and
    Medical Center
1015 N.W. 22nd Avenue
Suite 315
Portland, OR 97210
(503) 413-7540
www.legacyhealth.org

Northwest Sleep Health
Northwest Primary Care Group
13518 S.E. 97th Avenue
Clackamas, OR 97015
(503) 353-1272
www.nwsleephealth.com

PENNSYLVANIA

Bryn Mawr Hospital Sleep Medicine Services
The Bryn Mawr Hospital and Main
    Line Health
933 Haverford Road
Bryn Mawr, PA 19010
(610) 526-4305
www.mainlinesleep.com

Lehigh Valley Hospital Sleep Disorders Center
Lehigh Valley Hospital
17th & Chew Streets
P.O. Box 7017
Allentown, PA 18105-1707
(610) 402-9777
www.lvhhn.org

Sleep Disorders Center
Pennsylvania Hospital
800 Spruce Street
Third Floor, Spruce Building
Philadelphia, PA 19107
(215) 829-7079
www.pennhealth.com/pahosp/medicine/
  sleep.html

Sleep Research and Treatment Center
Milton S. Hershey Medical Center
500 University Drive
Hershey, PA 17033
(717) 531-8520
www.pennstatepsychiatry.com

RHODE ISLAND
Sleep Disorders Center of Lifespan Hospitals–Rhode Island Hospital
70 Catamore Boulevard
Providence, RI 02914
(401) 431-5420

SOUTH CAROLINA
Roper Sleep/Wake Disorders Center
Roper Hospital
316 Calhoun Street
Charleston, SC 29401-1125
(843) 724-2246
www.carealliance.com/sleep/index.html

SleepMed at South Carolina
1333 Taylor Street
Suite 6-B
Columbia, SC 29201
(803) 251-3093
www.sleepmed.md

Spartanburg Regional Medical Center Sleep Center
Spartanburg Regional Medical Center
101 E. Wood Street
Spartanburg, SC 29303
(864) 560-6904
www.srhs.com

SOUTH DAKOTA
Avera McKennan Sleep Diagnostic Center
Avera McKennan Hospital & University
  Health Center
Avera Doctor's Plaza 2
1100 E. 21st Street
Sioux Falls, SD 57117-5045
(605) 322-7378
www.mckennan.org

Sanford Medical Center Sleep Disorders Center
Sanford Medical Center
1621 S. Minnesota Avenue
Sioux Falls, SD 57117-5039
(605) 333-6302
www.sanfordhealth.org

The Sleep Center
Rapid City Regional Hospital
353 Fairmont Boulevard
Rapid City, SD 57701
(605) 719-8037
www.rcrh.com

TENNESSEE
Memorial North Park Sleep Center
Memorial North Park Hospital
2051 Hamill Road
Chattanooga, TN 37343
(423) 495-5297
www.memorial.org

Sleep Disorders Center
Erlanger Health System North Campus
632 Morrison Springs Road
Suite 300
Chattanooga, TN 37415
(423) 778-3316
www.erlanger.org

TEXAS

National Sleep Centers, Inc.
3500 Oakmont Boulevard
Suite 200
Austin, TX 78731
(512) 533-9400
www.nationalsleepcenters.com

The Sleep Center at Park Plaza
Park Plaza Hospital and Medical Center
1213 Hermann Drive
Lower Level #75
Houston, TX 77004
(713) 527-5337
www.parkplazahospital.com

Sleep Diagnostic Center–Beaumont
2627 Laurel Street
Beaumont, TX 77702
(409) 835-5382
sleepdiagnosticcenter.com

Sleep Medicine Institute
Presbyterian Hospital of Dallas
8200 Walnut Hill Lane
Jackson Building
Dallas, TX 75231
(214) 345-8563
www.sleepmed.com

Sonno Sleep Center
2311 N. Mesa
Building E
El Paso, TX 79902
(915) 533-8499
www.sonnosleep.com

UTAH

Advanced Research Systems/Pioneer Valley Sleep Disorders Center
Pioneer Valley Hospital
3336 S. 4155 W. #303
West Valley City, UT 84120
(801) 964-3876

Intermountain Sleep Disorders Center
LDS Hospital
8th Avenue & C Street
Salt Lake City, UT 84143
(801) 408-3618

Utah Sleep Medicine Center
1055 N. 300 W
Suite 402
Provo, UT 84604
(801) 357-7878

VERMONT

The Sleep Center at Rutland Regional Medical Center
Rutland Regional Medical Center
160 Allen Street
Rutland, VT 05701
(802) 747-3792
www.rrmc.org

VIRGINIA

RMH Center for Sleep Medicine
Rockingham Memorial Hospital
640 S. Main Street
Harrisonburg, VA 22801
(540) 437-8230

Sleep Disorders Center
Sentara Norfolk General Hospital/Eastern Virginia Medical School
600 Gresham Drive
Norfolk, VA 23507
(757) 388-2359
www.evms.edu/sleep/

Sleep Disorders Network
2955 Market Street
Suite B-1
Christiansburg, VA 24073
(540) 382-1165

WASHINGTON

Harrison Medical Center Sleep Disorders Center
2520 Cherry Avenue
Bremerton, WA 98310-4270
(360) 792-6686
www.harrisonmedical.org

NorthStar Sleep Center
NorthStar Medical Specialists
1345 King Street
Bellingham, WA 98229
(360) 676-1696
www.northstarmedicalspecialists.com

Pediatric Sleep Disorders Center
Childrens Hospital
1135 116th Avenue NE
Suite 420
Bellevue, WA 98004
(206) 987-8926
www.seattlechildrens.org

Sleep Center for Southwest Washington
Providence St. Peter Hospital
525 Lilly Road SE
Olympia, WA 98513
(360) 493-7686

WEST VIRGINIA

Charleston Sleep Diagnostics Laboratory
4500 MacCorkle Avenue SE
Charleston, WV 25304
(304) 254-9090

St. Mary's Regional Sleep Center
St. Mary's Hospital
2900 First Avenue
6th Floor East Wing
Huntington, WV 25702
(304) 526-1880
www.st-marys.org

The Weirton Sleep Center
Weirton Medical Center
651 Colliers Way
Suite 514
Weirton, WV 26062
(304) 797-6611
www.centerpointesleep.com

WISCONSIN

Bellin Sleep Center
Bellin Health System Hospital Center
744 S. Webster Avenue
Green Bay, WI 54301
(920) 433-7451
www.bellin.org

Sleep Disorders Center
Marshfield Clinic/St. Joseph's Hospital
2655 County Highway I
Chippewa Falls, WI 54729
(715) 726-4270
www.marshfieldclinic.org

Wisconsin Sleep Disorders Center Gundersen Clinic Ltd.
Gundersen Lutheran Medical Center
1910 South Avenue
La Crosse, WI 54601
(608) 775-2791
www.gundluth.org

In Canada

Additional centers can be found on http://sleepapnea.wikia.com/wiki/Canadian_Sleep_Labs

ALBERTA

Centre for Sleep and Human Performance
Suite 106-51 Sunpark Drive SE
Calgary, AB T2X 3V4
(403) 254-6663
www.centreforsleep.com

Sleep Medicine Program
Dept. of Psychiatry
University of Alberta
1Eb.14 Mackenzie Centre
University of Alberta Hospital
Edmonton, AB T6G 2B7
(780) 407-6565

BRITISH COLUMBIA

Sleep Disorders Program
UBC Hospital
2211 Westbrook Mall
Vancouver BC V6T 2B5
(604) 822-7606
www.vch.ca/sleep_disorders/

Sleep Surgery Centre, Inc.
303-2963 Glen Drive
Coquitlam, BC V3B 2P7
(604) 941-2344
www.sleepsurgerycentre.com

Vancouver Island Health Authority Sleep Lab
Royal Jubilee Hospital
1952 Bay Street
Victoria BC V8R 1J8
(250) 370-8008
http://www.viha.ca/respiratory_health/sleep_lab.htm

MANITOBA

Manitoba Sleep Disorders Centre
RS 303-810 Sherbrook Street
Winnipeg MB R3A 1R8
(294) 787-2063

RANA-Medical Respiratory Wellness Centre
#6-55 Henlow Bay
Winnipeg, MB R3 & 1G4
Hamilton ON L8P 4M3
(204) 928-1400
www.ranamedical.com/sleep

NEW BRUNSWICK

Atlantic Health Sciences Sleep Centre
Saint John Regional Hospital,
    400 University Avenue
Saint John, NB
(506) 648-6178
www.ahsc.health.nb.ca/Programs/MentalHealth/sleep.shtml

NEWFOUNDLAND & LABRADOR

St. Clare's Mercy Hospital Diagnostic Neurophysiology Sleep Lab
154 LeMarchant Road
St. John's NL A1C 5B8
(709) 777-5511
www.cdha.nshealth.ca

NOVA SCOTIA

Queen Elizabeth II Health Sciences Centre Sleep Disorders Laboratory and Clinic
Room 4005, AJLB, 4th Floor
5909 Veterans' Memorial Lane
Halifax NS B3H 2E2
(902) 473-4298
www.cdha.nshealth.ca

ONTARIO

The Centre for Sleep & Chronobiology
340 College Street
Suite 580
Toronto, ON M5T 3A9
(416) 603-9531
www.sleepmed.to

Cobourg Sleep Clinic
1060 Burnham Street
Unit 7
Cobourg, ON K9A 5V9
(905) 373-1227

Kingston General Hospital, Sleep Disorders Laboratory
Kingston General Hospital
Kidd 6 Room 22-6-005
76 Stuart Street
Kingston, ON K7L 2V7
(613) 548-6666 ext. 3347 or
    (613) 548-2382
http://www.kgh.on.ca/programs/sleep.asp

Niagara Snoring and Sleep Centre
6453 Morrison Street
Suite 204
Niagara Falls, ON L2E 7H1
(905) 374-2451

The Ottawa Hospital Sleep Centre, General Campus
501 Smyth Road
Ottawa, ON
(613) 737-8490

Royal Victoria Hospital
201 Georgian Drive
Barrie, ON L4M 6M2
(705) 728-9090 ext. 46238
www.rvh.on.ca

Royal Ottawa Hospital Sleep Disorders Service
1145 Carling Avenue
Ottawa, ON
613-722-6521 ext. 6248
www.rohcg.on.ca/sleep

Scarborough North Sleep Disorders Clinic
4040 Finch Avenue E
108
Scarborough, ON M1S 4V5
www.scarboroughsleepclinic.com

Sleep Disorders Clinic, Hamilton
Unit 7, 55 Frid Street
Hamilton, ON L8P 4M3
(905) 529 2259

Tri-Hospital Sleep Laboratory West
3024, Hurontario Street
Suite 208
Mississauga, ON L5B 4M4
(905) 566-1010
www.sleeplab.ca

QUÉBEC
Hôtel-Dieu de lévis
143 Wolfe
Lévis, QC, G6V 3Z1
(418) 835-7171

Laboratoire du sommeil/Sleep Laboratory
OSR Medical Inc./ Diagnostics Division
1361 Beaumont Avenue
Suite 202
Ville Mount-Royal, QC H3P 2H7
www.osrmedical.com

SASKATCHEWAN
Regina General Hospital
14401 14th Avenue
Regina, SK S4P 0W5
(306) 766-4444
www.rqhealth.ca

In the United Kingdom

Loughborough Sleep Research Centre
Loughborough University
Leicestershire
LE11 3TU
+44 1509 223091
http://www.lboro.ac.uk/departments/hu/
    groups/sleep/

Surrey Sleep Research Centre (SSRC)
Clinical Research Centre
Egerton Road
Guildford
Surrey
GU2 7XP
+44 1483 682502
http://www.surrey.ac.uk/SBMS/SSRC/

Department of Sleep Medicine, LUHD
The Royal Infirmary of Edinburgh
51 Little France Crescent
Old Dalkeith Road
Edinburgh
EH16 4SA
+44 131 242 3870
http://www.sleep.scot.nhs.uk/

In Australia

Centre for Sleep Research
Division of Education, Arts and Social
    Sciences
Level 7, Playford Building
University of South Australia
City East Campus
Frome Road
Adelaide SA 5000
+61 8 8302 6624
www.unisa.edu.au

Sleep and Circadian Group
Woolcock Institute of Medical Research
Level 3, Building 92
Royal Prince Alfred Hospital
Missenden Road
Camperdown NSW 2050
P.O. Box M77
Missenden Road NSW 2050
+61 2 9515 7546
www.woolcock.org.au

West Australian Sleep Disorders
    Research Institute
Internal Mailbox 201
Queen Elizabeth II Medical Centre
Hospital Avenue
Nedlands WA 6009
+61 8 9346 2422
www.wasdri.org.au

In New Zealand

Sleep/Wake Research Centre
Massey University
Ground Floor, 102 Adelaide Road
Newtown, Wellington
Private Bag 756, Wellington
+64 4 380 0603
www.sleepwake.massey.ac.nz

Acknowledgments

Every book is a collaboration of many minds—and this one is no exception.

I have had the generous cooperation and abundant support of an entire community of sleep researchers and the American Academy of Sleep Medicine. I am deeply grateful to the following for their intelligence, their work, and their willingness to share their knowledge with the rest of us:

David Dinges, Ph.D., visionary president of the World Federation of Sleep Research and Sleep Medicine Societies and chief of sleep and chronobiology at the University of Pennsylvania Medical School, gave me the intellectual framework within which to understand the studies of hundreds of researchers—and the cultural context in which to understand its potential impact upon my readers.

Cliff Saper, M.D., Ph.D., head of neurology at Harvard Medical School, carefully and patiently explained the finer points of flip switches, arm wrestling, and how the sleep strategies I gathered from sleep researchers influence the brain's complex circuitry and enable us to fall asleep.

Sonia Ancoli-Israel, Ph.D., a professor of psychiatry at the University of California at San Diego and a recent president of the Sleep Research Society, explained why our elders don't sleep, how light therapy works, and the importance of treating insomnia in those with depression.

Kathryn Lee, Ph.D., a sleep researcher at the University of California at San Francisco, sorted out how the complex milieu of women's hormones affect sleep at every biological life stage and offered practical strategies for each one.

Julie Silver, M.D., an assistant professor of physical medicine and rehabilitation at Harvard Medical School, not only contributed effective strategies to combat the effects of pain and cancer on sleep but pointed the way to people I needed to interview and studies I needed to see.

Ruth Benca, M.D., Ph.D., director of the sleep program at the University of Wisconsin-Madison, provided an insightful analysis of the relationship between insomnia and depression that offers the world a new way of looking at both.

Lawrence J. Epstein, M.D., recent president of the American Academy of Sleep Medicine and medical director of the Harvard-affiliated Sleep Health*Centers* in Brighton, Massachusetts, patiently parsed the intricacies of sleep medication and the effectiveness of cognitive behavioral therapy.

Mary S. Esther, M.D., president of the American Academy of Sleep Medicine, not only wrote the foreword for this book but also helped me understand how worry affects sleep.

Cathy A. Alessi, M.D., a professor at UCLA and associate director of clinical health services research at the Los Angeles Veterans Administration Healthcare System, helped me understand the major life stressors facing aging parents.

Margaret Moline, Ph.D., former head of the sleep center at Weill Cornell Medical College, pointed out the deleterious and wholly unconscious effect that access to information 24 hours a day has on sleep.

Celyne H. Bastien, Ph.D., a professor of psychology at the University of Laval in Quebec, pointed me to studies on the effectiveness of cognitive behavioral therapy online and on the phone.

Cecile Andrews, Ph.D., a groundbreaking thinker in simple living, offered down-to-earth concrete ways in which women could find both meaning and sleep in their lives.

Rebecca Gould, Ph.D., an associate professor studying simple-living practices at Middlebury College, articulated the challenge of bringing life and values into alignment so we can sleep.

Sara Mednick, Ph.D., a research scientist at the University of California at San Diego, detailed the life- and performance-enhancing benefits of napping.

Belleruth Naparstek, M.S., a gifted therapist, offered insight into grieving and helped me grasp both the shape of grieving and its weight.

JoAnn Manson, M.D., the Harvard researcher who pioneered much of the research that uncovered the dangers of hormone replacement therapy, explained the role HRT can play in perimenopausal sleep.

Frisca Yan-Go, M.D., medical director of the UCLA Sleep Disorders Center, detailed the effects of perimenopause on sleep and offered pragmatic strategies to overcome them.

Carolyn M. Kaelin, M.D., director of Harvard's Comprehensive Breast Health Center at Brigham and Women's Hospital, shared her own struggle to overcome breast cancer.

William H. Anderson, M.D., a member of the American Academy of Allergy, Asthma and Immunology, helped craft the anti-allergy sleep plan.

Kar-Ming Lo, M.D., FCCP, a critical-care specialist in the Summa Health System, explained how shift workers develop insomnia and how it could be overcome.

Grace Pien, M.D., a sleep researcher at the University of Pennsylvania's Center for Sleep and Respiratory Neurobiology, explained the surprisingly complex relationship between pregnancy and insomnia.

Jodi Mindell, Ph.D., associate director of the Sleep Center at the Children's Hospital of Philadelphia, helped craft our sleepless moms plan.

Donna Arand, Ph.D., clinical director of the Kettering Hospital Sleep Disorders Center in Dayton, Ohio, explained the effects of stress on sleep.

Jerilynn C. Prior, M.D., scientific director of the Center for Menstrual Cycle and Ovulation Research at the University of British Columbia, offered a framework within which to understand the hormonal roller coaster of perimenopause.

Eveline Honig, M.D., director of the Narcolepsy Network, contributed a plan to fight the effects of narcolepsy on sleep.

Kalyanakrishnan Ramakrishnan, M.D., an associate professor at the University of Oklahoma Health Sciences Center, was the first to make me aware that exercise improves sleep as effectively as drugs.

Becky Wang-Cheng, M.D., a medical director at Kettering Medical Center, explained the effect of temperature on the sleep of perimenopausal women and how we could counteract it.

Rochelle Goldberg, M.D., president of the American Sleep Apnea Association, helped craft our anti-apnea sleep plan.

James P. Krainson, M.D., a sleep medicine specialist at Miami's South Florida Sleep Diagnostic Center, pointed out the relationship between insomnia and depression.

George Niederehe, Ph.D., the National Institute of Mental Health's project officer for STAR *D, a nationwide series of studies on depression, clarified the effects of medication on depression.

Hrayr P. Attarian, M.D., director of the University of Vermont's regional sleep center and editor of the textbook *Sleep Disorders in Women*, recommended numerous researchers with whom I should talk.

Charles J. Bae, M.D., a sleep specialist at the Cleveland Clinic Sleep Disorders Center, helped me understand the effects of body temperature on sleep.

I also want to acknowledge the wonderful "sleepless" women from coast to coast who shared their stories and middle-of-the-night strategies throughout this book. I am humbled by their honesty.

But none of this would have been posssible without the dedication of the Reader's Digest staff. Julie Bain, health director of *Reader's Digest* magazine, who truly understands the needs of women on a gut level and who championed the need for a down-to-earth guide on sleep. My editor, Dolores York, who nurtured, supported, and championed the book, nipped at my heels when I might have drowned in a sea of data, and who was always ready to make the book better on every level.

On a personal note, my husband, Wayne, and my son, Matthew, kept me loved, sane, online, and technologically literate, while my friends Camille and Monica kept me swimming lap after lap after lap so that I might write and write and write. Finally, I would still be interviewing if it weren't for the help of my researcher Julie Evans, who even contributed a section of the book on breathing difficulties.

Thank you all so very, very much. I have been blessed by your generosity and care.

—Ellen Michaud

Index

Q

R

S